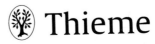

*For Claudia, with love and appreciation*

# Clinical Tests for the Musculoskeletal System

## Examinations—Signs—Phenomena

Klaus Buckup, MD
Klinikum Dortmund GmbH
Orthopedic Hospital
Dortmund, Germany

521 illustrations

2nd edition

Thieme
Stuttgart · New York

*Library of Congress Cataloging-in-Publication Data* is available from the publisher

This book is an authorized and revised translation of the 3rd German edition published and copyrighted 2005 by
Georg Thieme Verlag, Stuttgart, Germany. Title of the German edition: Klinische Tests an Knochen, Gelenken und Muskeln. Untersuchungen – Zeichen – Phänomene.

Translator: John Grossman MD, Schrepkow, Germany

Illustrators: Detlev Michaelis and Barbara Junghähnel

**Important note:** Medicine is an ever-changing science undergoing continual development. Research and clinical experience are continually expanding our knowledge, in particular our knowledge of proper treatment and drug therapy. Insofar as this book mentions any dosage or application, readers may rest assured that the authors, editors, and publishers have made every effort to ensure that such references are in accordance with **the state of knowledge at the time of production of the book.**
Nevertheless, this does not involve, imply, or express any guarantee or responsibility on the part of the publishers in respect to any dosage instructions and forms of applications stated in the book. **Every user is requested to examine carefully** the manufacturers' leaflets accompanying each drug and to check, if necessary in consultation with a physician or specialist, whether the dosage schedules mentioned therein or the contraindications stated by the manufacturers differ from the statements made in the present book. Such examination is particularly important with drugs that are either rarely used or have been newly released on the market. Every dosage schedule or every form of application used is entirely at the user's own risk and responsibility. The authors and publishers request every user to report to the publishers any discrepancies or inaccuracies noticed.

© 2008 Georg Thieme Verlag
Rüdigerstrasse 14, 70469 Stuttgart
Germany
http://www.thieme.de
Thieme New York, 333 Seventh Avenue,
New York, NY 10001 USA
http://www.thieme.com

Cover design: Thieme Publishing Group
Typesetting by primustype Hurler GmbH,
Notzingen, Germany
Printed in Germany by OAN, Zwenkau

ISBN 978-3-13-136792-1          1 2 3 4 5

# Preface

In view of the many investigative methods available, especially imaging techniques (digital radiography, ultrasound, CT, and MRI), some clinicians seem to forget the importance of a good examination—often to their detriment.

The experienced musculoskeletal physician, however, is aware of the wide range of interpretations associated with imaging findings. The evaluation of a genuine functional impairment and its significance is not easily achieved without corresponding clinical findings and tests. Therefore, clinical examination remains of key importance as the basis for a timely and accurate diagnosis. The popularity of the first edition of *Clinical Tests for the Musculoskeletal System* and the number of translated editions to date testify that this is not just a pious wish or assumption.

Nonetheless, anything can be improved upon. When one is satisfied and becomes complacent it does not take long to realize that others are already shifting gears and attempting to pass you by.

All chapters have been revised for the present edition. New tests are included, and suggestions from readers of previous editions have also been considered. To provide a better overview and to make diagnostic procedures easier, a synopsis in the form of a flow diagram has been included at the beginning of each chapter. This enhances the book's value as a reference work.

Many common special tests are tested for reliability. However, sometimes the validity of a test may be debatable. Each examiner is encouraged to use those tests he or she has found to be clinically effective. Under no circumstances should special tests be used in isolation. They should be viewed as an integral part of the total examination. Some new tests that I have included in this edition are based upon reader feedback, which indicates that these tests have gained in popularity.

Expanding upon my efforts in the first edition to provide reviewed literature for each test, I have performed an exhaustive search of the literature to include as much evidence as possible related to research carried out on each test. References are listed in the appendix.

In addition to referring to evidence-based, peer-reviewed papers, which evaluate the effectiveness of each test, I sometimes include additional comments and refer to other or similar clinical tests. This should help the reader to understand the historical or anatomical background of a test.

This new, updated edition is intended to facilitate the examination of our patients, in order to arrive at a diagnosis and initiate treatment more quickly.

I would like to thank Thieme Publishers Stuttgart, especially Dr. Clifford Bergman, Ms. Annie Hollins, and Ms. Elisabeth Kurz for the excellent cooperation.

Klaus Buckup

# Contents

# 1 Spine

Differential diagnosis of back pain is often a daunting task given the wide range of possible causes that must be considered. Terms such as "cervical spine syndrome" or "lumbar spine syndrome" are ambiguous as they identify neither the location nor the nature of the disorder.

Once the history has been taken, any examination of the spine should be preceded by a general physical examination. This is required to properly evaluate those changes in the spine that are attributable to causes elsewhere in the body such as in the limbs and muscles. The examination begins with inspection. General body posture is noted, and the position of the shoulders and pelvis (level of the shoulders, comparison of both shoulder blades, level of the iliac crests, lateral pelvic obliquity), vertical alignment of the spine (any deviation from vertical), and the profile of the back (kyphotic or lordotic deformity, or absence of physiologic kyphosis and/or lordosis) are evaluated. Palpation can detect changes in muscle tone such as contractures or myogelosis and can identify tender areas. The active and passive mobility of the spine as a whole and the mobility of specific segments are then evaluated.

In patients presenting with a spine syndrome, the first step is to identify the location and nature of the disorder. Tissue destruction, inflammation, and severe degenerative changes usually involve a characteristic clinical picture with corresponding radiographic and laboratory findings. A number of additional diagnostic modalities can supplement plain-film radiography in cases where further diagnostic studies are indicated to confirm or exclude a tentative diagnosis. The choice of additional imaging modalities depends on the line of inquiry. For example, computed tomography with its higher contrast between bone and soft tissue is more suitable for visualizing changes in bone than is magnetic resonance imaging, whose advantage lies in its high-resolution visualization of soft tissue. Dysfunctional muscular and ligamentous structures render the clinical evaluation of spine syndromes more difficult.

Radiographic and laboratory findings alone are rarely able to provide a conclusive diagnosis in these spinal disorders. This makes manual diagnostic techniques that focus on evaluation of function particularly important. The examiner evaluates changes in the skin (hyperalgesia and characteristics of the paraspinal skin fold, also known as Kibler fold), painful muscle spasms, painfully restricted mobility with loss of play in the joint, functional impairments with painful abnormal mobility, and radicular pain. The examination evaluates each part of the spine as a whole (cervical, thoracic, and lumbar) and each segment individually.

Because every pair of adjacent vertebrae is connected by many ligaments, only limited motion is possible in any one intervertebral joint. However, the sum of all the movements in the many vertebral articulations results in significant mobility in the spinal column and trunk as a whole. This mobility varies considerably between individuals (Fig. 1). The main motions are flexion and extension in the sagittal plane, lateral bending in the coronal plane, and rotation around the longitudinal axis. The cervical spine exhibits the greatest range of motion. It is both the most highly mobile portion of the spine and the one most susceptible to spinal disorders.

About 50% of flexion and extension occurs between the occiput and C1. The other 50% is distributed approximately evenly along the other cervical vertebrae, especially C5 and C6.

About 50% of rotation occurs between C1 (atlas) and C2 (axis). The other 50% is distributed evenly along the other five cervical vertebrae.

Rotation and lateral bending in the thoracic spine occur primarily in the lower thoracic spine and in the thoracolumbar junction. The lumbar spine with its sagittally aligned facet joints primarily allows flexion and extension (forward and backward bending) and lateral bending. The capacity for rotation is less well developed in this portion of the spine.

Neurologic examination can exclude sensory deficits and palsies of the lower extremities. This includes eliciting intrinsic reflexes to test for nerve stretching signs.

When examining the spine, the physician must consider the possibility that "back pain" may in fact be referred pain caused by pathology in other areas.

# Range of Motion of the Spine (Neutral-Zero Method)

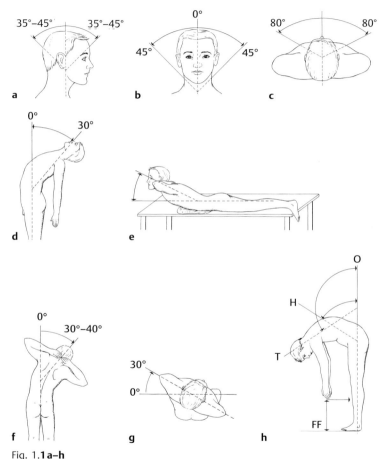

Fig. 1.**1a–h**
**a** Forward and backward bending (flexion and extension). **b** Lateral bending.
**c** Rotation in middle position 80/0/80°, rotation in flexion 45/0/45° (C0–C1),
rotation in extension 60/0/60°. **d, e** Backward bending (extension) of the spine:
standing (**d**) and prone (**e**). **f** Lateral bending of the spine. **g** Rotation of the trunk.
**h** Forward bending of entire spine: *H* flexion in hip, *T* total excursion, *FF* distance
between fingers and floor

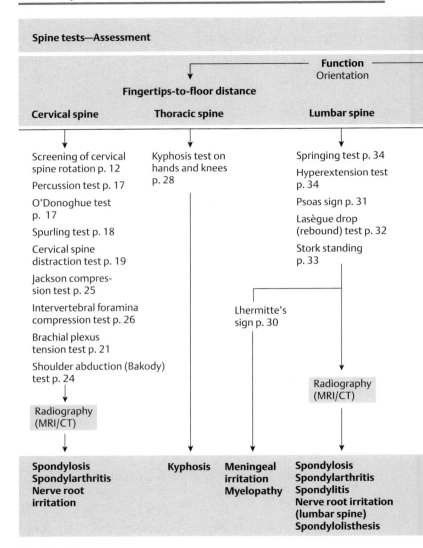

Fig. 1.2    Spine tests

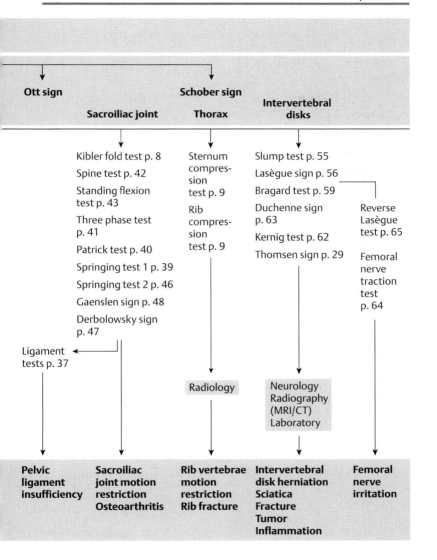

**Ott sign**

**Sacroiliac joint**

**Schober sign**

**Thorax**

**Intervertebral disks**

Kibler fold test p. 8
Spine test p. 42
Standing flexion test p. 43
Three phase test p. 41
Patrick test p. 40
Springing test 1 p. 39
Springing test 2 p. 46
Gaenslen sign p. 48
Derbolowsky sign p. 47

Sternum compression test p. 9
Rib compression test p. 9

Slump test p. 55
Lasègue sign p. 56
Bragard test p. 59
Duchenne sign p. 63
Kernig test p. 62
Thomsen sign p. 29

Reverse Lasègue test p. 65
Femoral nerve traction test p. 64

Ligament tests p. 37

Radiology

Neurology
Radiography (MRI/CT)
Laboratory

**Pelvic ligament insufficiency**

**Sacroiliac joint motion restriction
Osteoarthritis**

**Rib vertebrae motion restriction
Rib fracture**

**Intervertebral disk herniation
Sciatica
Fracture
Tumor
Inflammation**

**Femoral nerve irritation**

Table 1.1    Overview of general function tests of the spine

| |
|---|
| Fingertips-to-floor distance test |
| Ott sign |
| Schober sign |
| Neutral-zero method |

## Overview of Tests for Evaluating Spinal Function

1. Fingertips-to-floor distance test
2. Ott sign
3. Schober sign
4. Neutral-zero range of motion test (Fig. 1.1)

## Fingertips-to-Floor Distance Test in Flexion

Measures the mobility of the entire spine when bending forward (fingertip-to-floor distance in centimeters).

**Procedure:**  The patient is standing or seated on the examination table. When the patient bends over with the knees fully extended, both hands should come to rest at approximately the same distance from the feet. The distance between the patient's fingers and the floor is measured, or how far the patient's fingers reach may be recorded (knee, mid-tibia, etc.; Fig. **1 h**).

**Assessment:**  This mobility test assesses a combined motion involving both the hips and the spine. Good mobility in the hips can compensate for stiffening in the spine. In addition to the distance measured, the profile of the flexed spine should also be assessed (uniform kyphosis or fixed kyphosis).

A long distance between the fingertips and floor is therefore a nonspecific sign that is influenced by several factors:

1. Mobility of the lumbar spine
2. Shortening of the hamstrings
3. Presence of the Lasègue sign
4. Hip function

Clinically the fingertips-to-floor distance is used to assess the effect of treatment.

## Ott Sign

Measures the range of motion of the thoracic spine.

**Procedure:** The patient is standing. The examiner marks the C7 spinous process and a point 30 cm inferior to it. This distance increases by 2–4 cm in flexion and decreases by 1–2 cm in maximum extension (leaning backward).

**Assessment:** Degenerative inflammatory processes of the spine restrict spinal mobility and hence the range of motion of the spinous processes.

## Schober Sign

Measures the range of motion of the lumbar spine.

**Procedure:** The patient is standing. The examiner marks the skin above the S1 spinous process and a point 10 cm superior to it. These skin markings move up to about 15 cm apart in flexion and converge to a distance of 8–9 cm in maximum extension (leaning backward).

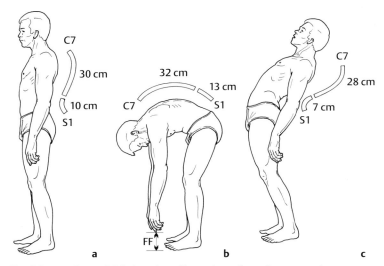

Fig. **1.3a–c** Ott and Schober signs (fingertip-to-floor distance test):
**a** upright position,
**b** flexion,
**c** extension

**Assessment:**   Degenerative inflammatory processes in the spine restrict spinal mobility and hence the range of motion of the spinous processes.

### Skin-Rolling Test (Kibler Fold Test)

Nonspecific back examination.

**Procedure:**   The patient lies prone with arms relaxed alongside the trunk. The examiner raises a fold of skin between thumb and forefinger and "rolls" it along the trunk or, on the extremities, perpendicular to the course of the dermatomes.

**Assessment:**   This test assesses regional variation in how readily the skin can be raised, the consistency of the skin fold (rubbery or edematous), and any lack of mobility in the skin. Palpation can detect regional tension in superficial and deep musculature as well as autonomic dysfunction (such as localized warming or increased sweating). In areas of hypalgesia, the skin is less pliable, more difficult to raise, and resists rolling. The patient reports pain. Areas of hypalgesia, tensed muscles, and autonomic dysfunction suggest vertebral disorders involving the facet joints or intercostal joints.

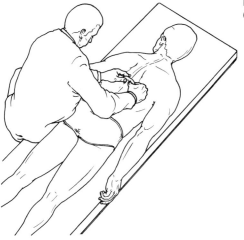

Fig. **1.4**   Skin-rolling test (Kibler fold test)

## ■ Chest Tests

### Sternum Compression Test

Indicates rib fracture.

**Procedure:** The patient is supine. The examiner exerts pressure on the sternum with both hands.

**Assessment:** Localized pain in the rib cage can be due to a rib fracture.
 Pain in the vicinity of the sternum or a vertebra suggests impaired costal or vertebral mobility.

### Rib Compression Test

Indicates impaired costovertebral or costosternal mobility or a rib fracture.

**Procedure:** The patient is seated. The examiner stands or crouches behind the patient and places his or her arms around the patient's chest, compressing it sagittally and horizontally.

**Assessment:** Compression of the rib cage increases the movement in the sternocostal and costotransverse joints and in the costovertebral

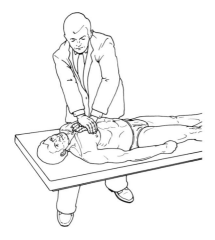

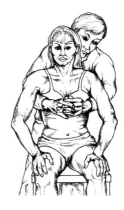

Fig. **1.5**   Sternum compression test          Fig. **1.6**   Rib compression test

joints. Performing the test in the presence of a motion restriction or other irritation in one of these joints elicits typical localized pain.

Pain along the body of a rib or between two ribs suggests a rib fracture or intercostal neuralgia.

## Chest Circumference Test

Measures the circumference of the chest at maximum inspiration and expiration.

**Procedure:**   The patient is standing or seated with arms hanging relaxed. The difference in chest circumference between maximum inspiration and expiration is measured. The circumference is measured immediately above the convexity of the breast in women, and immediately below the nipples in men.

The difference in chest circumference between maximum inspiration and expiration normally lies between 3.5 and 6 cm.

**Assessment:**   Limited depth of breathing is encountered in ankylosing spondylitis, where the impairment of inspiration and expiration is usually painless. Impaired or painful inspiration and expiration with limited depth of breathing is observed in costal and vertebral dysfunctions (motion restricted), inflammatory or tumorous pleural processes, and pericarditis. Bronchial asthma and emphysema are associated with painless impaired expiration.

## Schepelmann Test

For the differential diagnosis of chest pain.

**Procedure:**   The patient is seated and is asked to bend first to one side, then to the other.

**Assessment:**   Pain on the concave side is a sign of intercostal neuralgia; If pain occurs on the convex side, the diagnosis is intercostal myofascitis. Intercostal myofascitis must be differentiated from the fibrous inflammation of pleurisy. Rib fractures are painful on any movement of the spine.

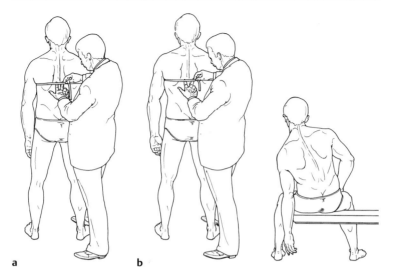

Fig. **1.7a, b** Chest circumference test:
**a** at maximum expiration,
**b** at maximum inspiration

Fig. **1.8** Schepelmann test

## ■ Cervical Spine Tests

### Cervical Spine—Range Of Motion—Screening (ROM)

The ROM available in the cervical spine is the sum of the ranges of motion between the head and C1 and any pair of vertebrae as part of the cervical spine. Many factors can influence this ROM: These include flexibility of the intervertebral disks, shape and inclination of the articular processes of the facet joints, and the degree of laxity of the ligaments and joint capsules.

Except in flexion females tend to have a greater active ROM than males.

The ROM decreases with age. However, the range of rotation between C1 and C2 may increase with age.

The passive ROM with the patient supine is normally greater than the active and passive ROM with the patient sitting. This can be explained by the fact that in the sitting position the head has to be held up against gravity, which is achieved by increased muscular tension preventing excessive motion in the neck and spine.

For this reason passive movements with overpressure should always be performed along with active movements, whereas active movements with overpressure at the end of the range do not give a true impression of the endpoint of motion in the cervical spine. If passive movements with overpressure are normal and pain free, the examiner may test the quadrant position carefully.

The quadrant position is end-range extension, lateral flexion, and rotation. This stresses the anterior, posterior, and lateral tissues of the neck including the vertebral artery. Overpressure can cause various symptoms in this position. This is highly suggestive of: (a) nerve root pathology (radicular signs), (b) apophyseal joint involvement (localized pain), and (c) vertebral artery involvement (dizziness, nausea).

## Screening of Cervical Spine Rotation

**Procedure:**  The patient is seated and upright. The examiner holds the patient's head with both hands around the parietal region and, with the patient's neck slightly extended, passively rotates the patient's head to one side and then the other from the neutral position.

**Assessment:**  The range of motion is determined by comparing both sides. The examiner also notes quality of the endpoint of motion, which is resilient in normal conditions but hard when functional impairment is present.

Restricted mobility with pain is a sign of segmental dysfunction (arthritis, blockade, inflammation, or muscle shortening). Restricted rotation with a hard endpoint and pain at the end of the range of motion suggest degenerative changes, predominately in the middle cervical vertebrae (spondylosis, spondylarthritis, or uncovertebral arthritis).

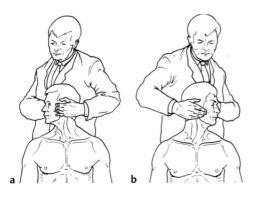

Fig. **1.9a, b**  Screening of cervical spine rotation:
**a** at maximum right rotation,
**b** at maximum left rotation

A soft endpoint is more probably attributable to shortening of the long extensors of the neck or the longus colli muscle.

**Note:** The vertebral arteries may be compressed as a result of chronic degenerative disease of the cervical spine. Rotating the head causes compression of the vertebral arteries. Vertigo, nausea, dizziness, visual disturbance, syncope, and nystagmus are all signs of buckling of the ipsilateral vertebral artery (Barré–Liéou sign). The patient with a positive Barré–Liéou sign is a poor candidate for aggressive cervical spine manipulation.

### Test of Head Rotation in Maximum Extension

Functional test of the lower cervical spine.

**Procedure:** The patient is seated. Holding the back of the patient's head with one hand and the patient's chin with the other, the examiner passively extends the patient's neck (tilts the head backwards) and

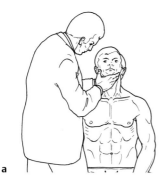

a

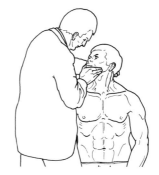

b

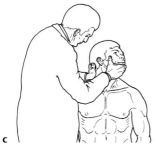

c

Fig. **1.10a–c** Test of head rotation in maximum extension:
**a** backward tilt,
**b** right rotation,
**c** left rotation

rotates the head to both sides. This motion involves slight lateral bending in the cervical spine.

**Assessment:**  In maximum extension, the region of the atlantooccipital joint is locked and rotation largely takes place in the lower segments of the cervical spine and in the cervicothoracic junction. Restricted mobility with pain is a sign of segmental dysfunction. The most likely causes include degenerative changes in the middle and lower cervical spine (spondylosis, spondylarthritis, or uncovertebral arthritis). Vertigo suggests compromised vascular supply from the vertebral artery.

### Test of Head Rotation in Maximum Flexion

Functional test of the upper cervical spine.

**Procedure:**  The patient is seated. Holding the back of the patient's head with one hand and the patient's chin with the other, the examiner passively flexes the patient's neck (tilts the head forward) and rotates

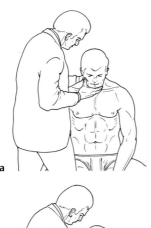

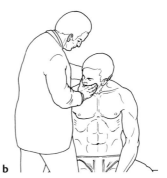

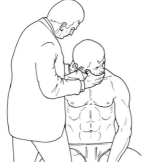

Fig. **1.11a–c**   Test of head rotation in maximum flexion:
**a**  forward tilt,
**b**  right rotation,
**c**  left rotation

the head to both sides. This motion involves slight lateral bending in the cervical spine.

**Assessment:**  In maximum flexion, the segments below C2 are locked and rotation largely takes place in the atlantooccipital and atlantoaxial joints. Restricted mobility with pain is a sign of segmental dysfunction. The most likely causes to consider include degenerative causes, instability, and inflammatory changes. Any occurrence of autonomic symptoms such as vertigo require further diagnostic studies.

## Test of Segmental Function in the Cervical Spine

**Procedure and assessment:**  For direct diagnostic testing of segmental function in the cervical spine, the examiner stands next to the patient. Placing one hand around the patient's head so that his or her elbow is front of the patient's face, the examiner then places the ulnar edge of the same hand with the little finger on the arch of the upper vertebra of the segment to be examined. Segmental mobility is evaluated with the palpating finger of the contralateral hand. Posterior and lateral mobility in the segment can be assessed by applying slight traction with the upper hand. Rotation in the segment can also be evaluated during the same examination.

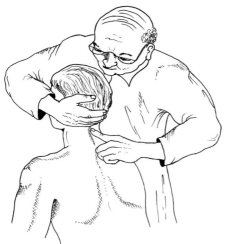

Fig. **1.12**   Test of segmental function in the cervical spine

For diagnostic testing of segmental function in the cervicothoracic junction in flexion and extension, the examiner immobilizes the patient's head with one hand and places the fingers of the other hand on the three adjacent spinous processes. By passively flexing and extending the patient's neck, the examiner can assess the range of motion in the individual segments by observing the excursion of the spinous processes.

### Soto–Hall Test

Nonspecific test of cervical spine function.

**Procedure:**  The patient is supine and first actively raises his or her head slightly to bring the chin as close as possible to the sternum. The examiner then passively tilts the patient's head forward, at the same time exerting light pressure on the sternum with the other hand.

**Assessment:**  Pain in the back of the neck when pressure is applied during passive raising of the head suggests a bone or ligament disorder in the cervical spine. Pulling pain occurring when the patient actively raises the neck is primarily due to shortening of the posterior neck musculature.

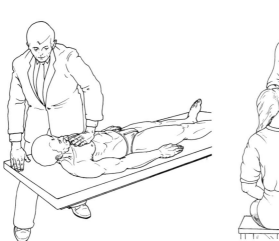

Fig. 1.**13**   Soto–Hall test

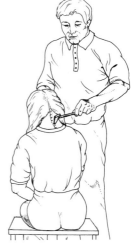

Fig. 1.**14**   Percussion test

## Percussion Test

**Procedure:** With the patient's cervical spine slightly flexed, the examiner taps the spinous processes of all the exposed vertebrae.

**Assessment:** Localized nonradicular pain is a sign of a fracture or of muscular or ligamentous functional impairment. Radicular symptoms indicate intervertebral disk pathology with nerve root irritation.

## O'Donoghue Test

Differentiates between ligamentous pain and muscular pain in the back of the neck.

**Procedure:** The seated patient's head is passively tilted first to one side and then the other. Then the patient is asked to tilt his or her head to one side against the resistance of the examiner's hand resting on the zygomatic bone and temple.

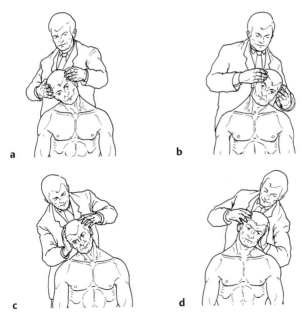

Fig. 1.**15a–d**   O'Donoghue test:
**a, b** passive motion,
**c, d** active motion against resistance

**Assessment:**   Occurrence of pain during this active head motion with isometric tensing of the ipsilateral and contralateral paravertebral musculature suggests muscular dysfunction, whereas pain during passive lateral bending of the cervical spine suggests a functional impairment involving ligaments or articular, possibly degenerative processes.

## Valsalva Test

**Procedure:**   The patient is seated with the thumb in the mouth and attempts to push the thumb out by blowing out hard.

**Assessment:**   The pushing increases the intraspinal pressure, revealing the presence of space-occupying masses such as extruded intervertebral disks, tumors, narrowing due to osteophytes, and soft tissue swelling. This leads to radicular symptoms entirely confined to the respective dermatome or dermatomes.

   The test should be performed with great caution, because the patient may lose consciousness during the test or afterward. The mechanism can block the blood supply to the brain. Test results are very subjective.

## Spurling Test

Assesses facet joint pain and nerve root irritation.

**Procedure:**   The patient is seated with the head rotated and tilted to one side. The patient bends or laterally flexes the head to the unaffected side first, then to the affected side. With the other hand, the examiner lightly taps (compresses) the hand resting on the patient's head. If the patient tolerates this initial step of the test, it is then repeated with the cervical spine extended as well.

**Assessment:**   If pain radiates from the cervical spine down the patient's arm the test is considered to be positive.

   Simultaneous extension of the cervical spine narrows the intervertebral foramina by 20–30%.

   In conditions such as cervical stenosis, spondylosis, osteophytes, trophic facet joints, or herniated disks, the foramina may already be smaller then normal.

   The test is not considered to be positive if neck pain only is present, without radiation into the shoulder or arm.

   If the pain and an altered sensation can be localized in the area of a certain dermatome, this can possibly indicate which nerve root is involved.

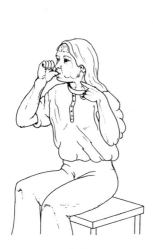

Fig. 1.**16** Valsalva test

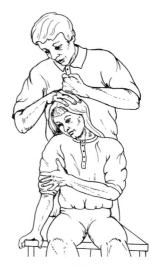

Fig. 1.**17** Spurling test

Conditions like myalgia, whiplash syndromes, etc. can cause increased muscular tension. Pain can be felt on the opposite side to where the head is bent. This is called a reverse Spurling sign and is indicative of muscle spasm.

**Note:** Pain on the concave side indicates nerve root or facet joint pathology (Spurling sign). Pain on the convex side indicates muscle strain (reverse Spurling sign).

The Spurling test is an aggressive cervical compression test and the patient should be informed of each step as it is introduced.

The test should not be performed where a cervical fracture, dislocation, or instability are suspected or cannot be ruled out.

### Cervical Spine Distraction Test

Differentiates between radicular pain in the back of the neck, shoulder, and arm and ligamentous or muscular pain in these regions.

**Procedure:** The patient is seated. The examiner grasps the patient's head about the jaw and the back of the head and applies superior axial traction.

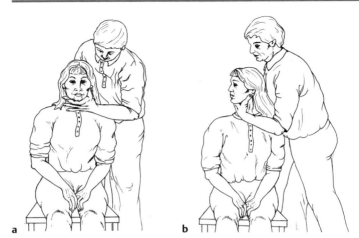

Fig. 1.**18a, b**   Cervical spine distraction test:
**a** middle position,
**b** rotation

**Assessment:**   Distraction of the cervical spine reduces the load on the intervertebral disks and exiting nerve roots within the affected levels or segments while producing a gliding motion in the facet joints. Reduction of radicular symptoms, even in passive rotation, when the cervical spine is distracted is a sign of discogenic nerve root irritation. Increased pain during distraction and rotation suggests a functional impairment in the cervical spine due to muscular or ligamentous pathology or articular, possibly degenerative processes.

**Note:** The procedure not only indicates the nature of the patient's complaint, but also identifies the merit of cervical traction in the treatment regimen.

### Shoulder Press Test

**Procedure:**   The patient is seated and the examiner presses downward on one shoulder while bending the cervical spine laterally toward the contralateral side. This test is always performed on both sides.

**Assessment:**   Provocation of radicular symptoms is a sign of adhesion of the dural sac and/or a nerve root. If the pain is increased during the test, this indicates irritation or compression of the nerve roots, foraminal narrowing by osteophytes, adhesions around the dural sheath of

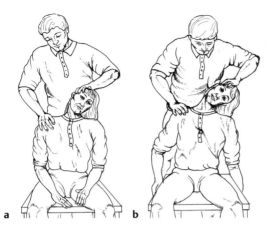

Fig. 1.**19a, b**
Shoulder press test:
**a** lateral bending,
**b** forced lateral
bending

the nerve and adjacent joint capsules, or a hypomobile joint capsule on the side being tested. Circumscribed pain on the side of the stretched musculature indicates increased muscle tone in the sternocleidomastoid or trapezius. Decreased muscular pain in the side that is not stretched suggests a pulled muscle or a functional impairment involving shortening of the musculature.

## Brachial Plexus Tension Test

Brachial plexus lesions result in motor and sensory syndromes of muscles of the upper extremities.

**Procedure:** The sitting patient abducts and then externally rotates the arms until symptoms occur. Then the patient lowers the arms until symptoms disappear. The examiner fixes the patient's arm in this position. While the shoulders are supported in position, the patient flexes the elbows and places the hands behind the head.

**Assessment:** If reproduction of symptoms can be created by flexion of the elbow the test is positive. The ulnar nerve and the C8 and T1 nerve roots are tested primarily. Flexing the cervical spine as well will increase symptoms.

**Note:** With the arm held upward and backward and the elbow fully flexed, the patient extends the shoulder and then the elbow. If radicular pain results, then the test is positive (Bikele sign) for a brachial plexus lesion.

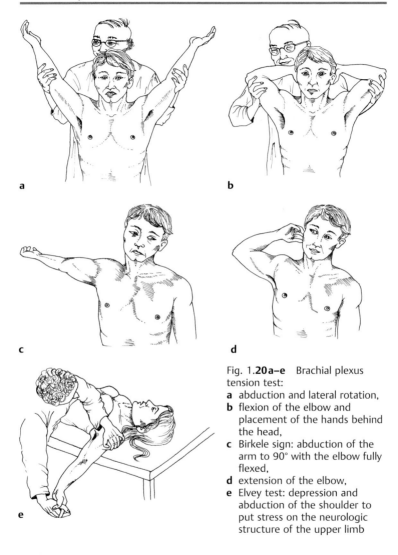

Fig. 1.**20a–e**   Brachial plexus tension test:
**a**  abduction and lateral rotation,
**b**  flexion of the elbow and placement of the hands behind the head,
**c**  Birkele sign: abduction of the arm to 90° with the elbow fully flexed,
**d**  extension of the elbow,
**e**  Elvey test: depression and abduction of the shoulder to put stress on the neurologic structure of the upper limb

The brachial plexus tension test is a modification of the upper limb tension test (Elvey test). They are tension tests designed to put stress on the neurologic structures of the upper limb. Modification and the posi-

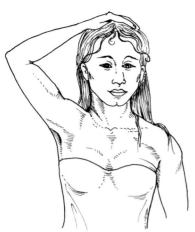

Fig. 1.**21**   Shoulder abduction (Bakody) test: the hand is placed on top of the head

tion of the shoulder, elbow, forearm, wrist, and fingers places greater stress on specific nerves.

When positioning the shoulder it is essential that a constant depression force be applied to the shoulder girdle so that, even with abduction the shoulder girdle remains depressed.

While the shoulder girdle is depressed the glenohumeral joint is taken to the appropriate abduction position (110° or 10° depending on the test), and the forearm, wrist, and fingers are taken to their appropriate end-of-range position.

**Test 1:**   Shoulder abduction 110°, elbow extension, forearm supination, wrist extension, finger and thumb extension.

Nerve bias—median nerve, anterior interosseous nerve, C5/C6/C7.

**Test 2:**   Shoulder abduction 10°, elbow extension, forearm supination, wrist extension, finger and thumb extension, shoulder lateral rotation.

Nerve bias—median nerve, musculocutaneous nerve, axillary nerve.

**Test 3:**   Shoulder abduction 10°, elbow extension, forearm pronation, wrist flexion and ulnar deviation, finger and thumb flexion, shoulder medial rotation.

Nerve bias—radial nerve.

**Test 4:**   Shoulder abduction—10° to 90°, hand to ear (Bikele sign), elbow flexion, forearm supination, wrist extension and radial deviation, finger and thumb extension, shoulder lateral rotation.

Nerve bias—ulnar nerve, C8 and T1 nerve roots.

## Shoulder Abduction (Bakody) Test

This test demonstrates involvement of nerve roots C4 or C5.

**Procedure:**  The patient is seated or supine while the examiner passively or the patient actively places the palm of the affected arm on the top of the head.

**Assessment:**  Cervical extradural compression by a herniated disk, epidural vein compression or nerve root compression, usually C4–C5 or C5–C6, can be shown by a decrease in or relief of symptoms. The roots can be determined by the distribution of the symptoms to specific dermatomes. This is also called the Bakody sign.

Abduction of the arm decreases the length of the nerve and decreases the tension of the lower nerve roots. If the pain increases with the positioning of the arm as described above, this implies that pressure increases in the interscalene triangle during testing. Patients with moderate to severe radicular symptoms usually do not have to be directed into the Bakody sign position, because it also is an antalgic posture that relieves pain.

## Test of Maximum Compression of the Intervertebral Foramina

**Procedure:**  The seated patient actively rotates his or her head to one side while slightly extending the neck.

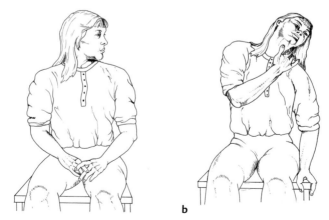

**a**

**b**

Fig. 1.**22a, b**   Test of maximum compression of the intervertebral foramina:
**a** rotation (start position),
**b** rotation and extension

**Assessment:** This pattern of motion leads to compression of the intervertebral foramina with narrowing of the intervertebral spaces and irritation of the nerve roots with corresponding radicular pain symptoms.

Occurrence of local pain without distal radicular symptoms in the dermatome concerned will be attributable to facet joint dysfunction. Pain on the convex side indicates muscular strain.

### Jackson Compression Test

**Procedure:** The patient is seated. The examiner stands behind the patient with his or her hand on the top of the patient's head and passively tilts the head to either side. In maximum lateral bending, the examiner presses down on the head to exert axial pressure on the spine. The head is slightly rotated to the involved side.

**Assessment:** The axial loading results in increased compression of the intervertebral disks, exiting nerve roots, and facet joints. Pressure on the intervertebral foramina acts on the facet joints to elicit distal pain that does not exactly follow identifiable segmental dermatomes. Presence of nerve root irritation will cause radicular pain symptoms. Local circumscribed pain will be attributable to stretching of the contralateral musculature of the neck.

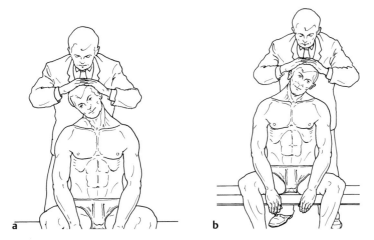

Fig. 1.**23a, b**  Jackson compression test:
**a**  right lateral bending,
**b**  left lateral bending

## Intervertebral Foramina Compression Test

**Procedure:**   Axial compression is applied to the cervical spine in the neutral (0°) position.

**Assessment:**   Compression of the intervertebral disks and exiting nerve roots, the facet joints, and/or the intervertebral foramina increases a radicular, strictly segmental pattern of symptoms. The presence of diffuse symptoms that are not clearly specific to any one segment may be regarded as a sign of ligamentous or articular functional impairment (facet joint pathology).

## Flexion Compression Test

**Procedure:**   The patient is seated. The examiner stands behind the patient and passively moves the cervical spine into flexion (tilts the patient's head forward). Then axial compression is applied to the top of the head.

**Assessment:**   This is a good test of the integrity of the intervertebral disk. In the presence of a posterolateral disk extrusion, this maneuver will press the extruded portion of the disk in a posterior direction, resulting in increasing compression of the nerve root. An increase in radicular symptoms can therefore indicate the presence of a posterolateral disk extrusion.

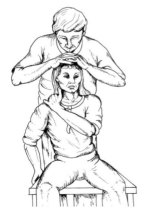

Fig. 1.**24**   Intervertebral foramina compression test

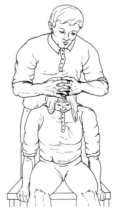

Fig. 1.**25**   Flexion compression test

The forward tilting of the head usually reduces the load on the facet joints and can reduce pain due to degenerative changes. Increasing pain may indicate an injury to posterior ligamentous structures.

### Extension Compression Test

**Procedure:** The patient is seated and the examiner stands behind the patient. The cervical spine is extended 30°. The examiner then applies axial compression to the top of the head.

**Assessment:** This test assesses the integrity of the intervertebral disk. Where a posterolateral extrusion with an intact annulus fibrosus is present, shifting the pressure on the disks anteriorly will reduce symptoms. Increased pain without radicular symptoms usually indicates an irritation in the facet joints as a result of decreased mobility due to degenerative changes.

## ■ Thoracic Spine Tests

Thoracic spinal pain may arise from somatic or visceral origins. Pain felt along the thoracic spine may arise from the ribs, the abdomen, or the spinal column.

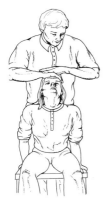

Fig. 1.**26**   Extension compression test

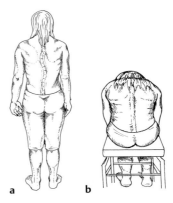

Fig. 1.**27a, b**   Adams forward bend test:
**a** upright posture,
**b** forward bending

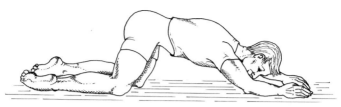

Fig. 1.**28**   Kyphosis test on hands and knees

## Adams Forward Bend Test

Assesses structural or functional scoliosis.

**Procedure:**   The patient is seated or standing. The examiner stands behind the patient and asks the patient to bend forward.

**Assessment:**   This test is performed in patients with detectable scoliosis of uncertain etiology or as a screening examination in patients with a family history of scoliotic posture. If the scoliotic posture improves during forward bending, then the condition is a functional scoliosis; where the scoliotic deformity remains with the same projection of the ribs and the lumbar distortion observed in upright posture, the condition is true scoliosis with structural changes.

## Kyphosis Test on Hands and Knees

**Procedure:**   The patient is asked to kneel down and stretch out his or her arms as far forward as possible on the floor.

**Assessment:**   This posture will correct a flexible kyphotic deformity of the thoracic spine. A kyphotic posture that remains unchanged is a fixed deformity.

## Test of Segmental Function in the Thoracic Spine in Extension and Flexion

**Procedure:**   The seated patient clasps both hands behind his or her head with the elbows together. The examiner immobilizes the patient's arms in front of the patient with one hand, leaving the examining hand free.

**Assessment:**   The examiner can detect segmental functional impairments by palpating the individual segments while passively moving the

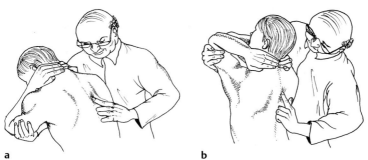

Fig. 1.**29a, b**   Test of segmental function in the thoracic spine:
**a** flexion,
**b** extension

patient's spine into flexion, extension, lateral bending, and rotation. A similar technique can also be used to evaluate segmental function in the lumbar spine.

## ■ Lumbar Spine Tests

Back pain is the most prevalent human affliction. Most patients have a mechanical cause (muscle strain, osteoarthritis, or disk tear) for their back pain. Lower back pain is frequently associated with sciatica problems.

### Thomsen Sign—Prone Knee Flexion Test

**Procedure:**   The patient lies prone and the examiner passively flexes the knee to maximum, so that the patient's heel touches the buttock. The examiner should make sure that the patient's hip is not rotated. If the examiner cannot flex the patient's knee to 90° due to a pathologic condition in the hip the test may be performed with passive extension of the hip while the knee is kept flexed as much as possible.

**Assessment:**   Unilateral neurologic pain in the lumbar area, buttock, and posterior thigh can indicate L2 or L3 nerve root lesions. During this test the femoral nerve will also be stretched. Pain occurring in the anterior thigh indicates tight quadriceps muscles or stretching of the femoral nerve.

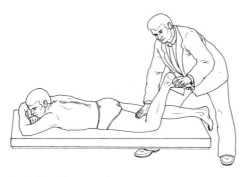

Fig. 1.**30**   Thomsen sign

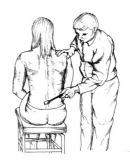

Fig. 1.**31**   Spinous process tap test

### Spinous Process Tap Test

Indicates lumbar spine syndrome.

**Procedure:**  The patient is seated with the spine slightly flexed. With a reflex mallet, the examiner taps on the spinous processes of the lumbar spine and on the paraspinal musculature.

**Assessment:**  Localized pain can indicate irritation of the involved spinal segments as a result of degenerative inflammatory changes. Radicular pain can be a sign of disk pathology.

### Lhermitte's Sign

Evaluation of spinal cord and upper motor neuron lesions.

**Procedure:**  The patient is sitting on the examining table with his legs straight.
The examiner passively flexes the patient's head and one hip simultaneously with the leg kept straight.

**Assessment:**  The test is positive when sharp pain radiates down the spine and into the upper or lower limbs. This indicates dural or meningeal irritation within the spine or possibly cervical myelopathy.
If the patient has to flex the head actively to the chest while lying supine the test is called the Soto Hall test. Flexing the hip to 130° places greater traction on the spinal cord.

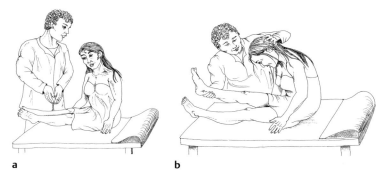

Fig. 1.**32a, b** Lhermitte's sign:
**a** sitting upright, legs outstretched,
**b** simultaneous flexion of the head and hip

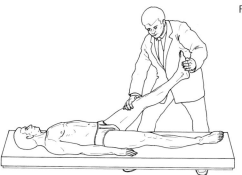

Fig. 1.**33** Psoas sign

## Psoas Sign

For diagnostic assessment of lumbar pain.

**Procedure:** The patient is supine and raises one leg with the knee extended. The examiner presses suddenly on the anterior aspect of the thigh.

**Assessment:** This sudden pressure on the distal thigh causes reflexive contraction of the iliopsoas with traction on the transverse processes of the lumbar spine. Patients will report pain in the presence of disorders in the lumbar spine (spondylarthritis, spondylitis, or disk herniation) or in the sacroiliac joint.

## Lasègue Drop (Rebound) Test

Differentiates lumbar pain.

**Procedure:**   The patient is supine. The examiner performs a straight-leg raising test until the patient begins to feel discomfort, then the examiner lets go of the leg from this position.

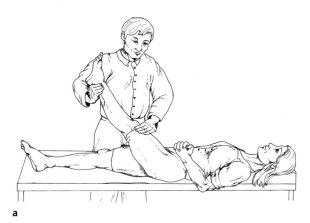

a

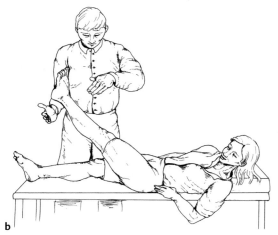

b

Fig. 1.**34a, b**   Lasègue straight leg drop test:
**a**  raising the leg,
**b**  dropping the leg

**Assessment:** Suddenly and unexpectedly letting go of the leg precipitates reflexive contraction of the muscles of the back and buttocks. It is primarily the iliopsoas that contracts, placing traction on the transverse processes of the lumbar spine. Patients will report pain in the presence of disorders of the lumbar spine (spondylarthritis, spondylitis, or disk herniation) or disorders of the sacroiliac joints (see psoas sign).

For a differential diagnosis it must be borne in mind that this test can also intensify visceral pain such as that caused by appendicitis.

### One-Leg Standing (Stork Standing), Lumbar Extension Test

Evaluation of joint dysfunction.

**Procedure:** The patient stands on one leg and extends the spine while balancing on that leg. The test is repeated with the patient standing on the opposite leg.

**Assessment:** The test is positive if back pain occurs. This can be associated with an interarticular stress fracture in spondylolisthesis. If the stress fracture is unilateral, standing on the leg of the affected side

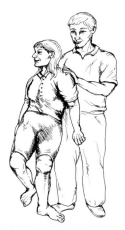

Fig. 1.**35** Standing on one leg (Stork position), lumbar extension test: Standing on one leg and extending the spine while balancing on the leg

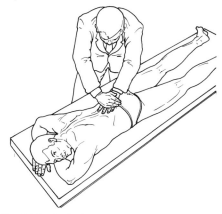

Fig. 1.**36** Springing test

causes more pain. If pain occurs on extension combined with rotation this is an indicator of possible facet joint pathology on the side to which the spine is rotated.

## Lumbar Spine Springing Test

For localization of functional impairments in the lumbar spine.

**Procedure:**   The patient is prone. The examiner palpates the articular processes or laminae of the vertebrae in question with his or her index and middle fingers. With the ulnar edge of the other hand, which is held perpendicularly over the palpating fingers, the examiner repeatedly presses lightly in a posteroanterior direction. The palpating fingers conduct this light springing pressure to the articular processes or laminae of the vertebrae in question.

**Assessment:**   Where joint function is intact, the articular processes or laminae will be resilient.

Lack of or excessive resiliency is a sign of abnormal segmental mobility, in the former case a blockade and in the latter case hypermobility. However, this test is also a provocative test for the posterior longitudinal ligament in particular and will result in an increase in the deep, dull low back pain that is typical of this structure and is difficult to localize.

## Hyperextension Test

Indicates a lumbar spine syndrome.

**Procedure:**   The patient is prone. The examiner immobilizes both the patient's legs and asks the patient to raise his or her torso.

In the second phase of the examination, the examiner passively extends the patient's spine and adds a rotational motion. The examiner's other hand rests on the patient's lumbar spine and is used to assess both the mobility in the lumbar spine and the level of the painful site.

**Assessment:**   Where segmental dysfunction in the lumbar spine is present, active extension of the lumbar spine will elicit or increase pain. The passive extension with an additional rotational motion allows the examiner to assess diminished segmental and/or regional mobility. A hard endpoint of the range of motion suggests degenerative changes, whereas a soft endpoint more probably suggests shortening of the longissimus thoracis and iliocostalis lumborum.

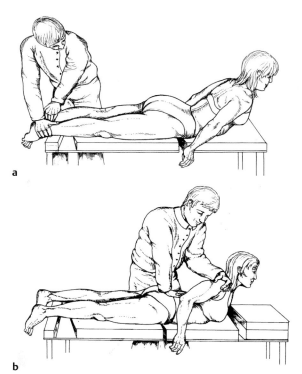

Fig. 1.**37a, b**  Hyperextension test:
**a** active hyperextension,
**b** passive hyperextension and rotation

## Supported Forward Bend Test (Belt Test)

Differentiates lumbar pain from iliosacral pain.

**Procedure:**  The patient is standing. The examiner stands behind the patient and asks the patient to bend forward until lumbosacral pain is felt. The patient then returns to the upright position. The examiner again asks the patient to bend forward. This time the examiner supports the patient's sacrum with his or her thigh and guides the motion by grasping both ilia.

**Assessment:**  Forward bending requires normal function in the sacroiliac joint and the lumbosacral junction as well as mobility in the indi-

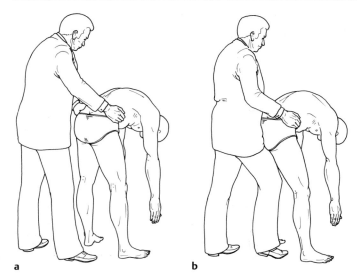

Fig. 1.**38a, b**   Supported forward bend test:
**a**  forward bending without support,
**b**  supported forward bending

vidual segments of the lumbar spine. Pain in unguided motion suggests a sacroiliac syndrome; this pain will improve or disappear in guided motion with the pelvis immobilized.

Changes in the lumbar spine will produce pain in forward bending with or without support.

### Sacroiliac Joint

The sacrum forms the base of the spine and is connected to the two halves of the pelvis (the ilia) by articulations known as the sacroiliac joints. While these articulations are true joints in the anatomic sense, from a functional standpoint they may be regarded as symphyses: the tight ligaments surrounding the bone and the crescentic shape and uneven contour of the articular surfaces effectively minimize mobility in these joints. In spite of this, compensatory movements between the spine and pelvis can result in significant impairments in this joint that can eventually affect the entire spine and the joints of the lower extremities.

Table 1.2  Function and provocation tests of the sacroiliac joint

Mennell sign

Springing test

Mobilization test

Standing flexion test

Variable leg length

Spine test

Patrick test (fabere test)

Three-phase hyperextension test

Motion restriction or instability of a sacroiliac joint can develop secondary to trauma, dislocation, or pelvic fractures. However, they may also develop as a result of asymmetrical loads on the pelvis or for other reasons. Pain during motion will be felt in the sacroiliac, gluteal, inguinal, and trochanteric regions. Usually it will radiate posteriorly within the S1 dermatome as far as the knee, occasionally producing symptoms resembling sciatica. Often patients will also experience pain in the lower abdomen and groin due to tension in the iliopsoas. Sacroiliac joint symptoms usually manifest themselves as tenderness to palpation and tapping in the parasacral region adjacent to the sacroiliac joints. A number of manipulative tests may be performed on the standing, supine, or prone patient to identify functional impairments in the sacroiliac joints.

## Ligament Tests

Functional assessment of the pelvic ligaments.

**Procedure:**  The patient is prone.

a) To evaluate the iliolumbar ligament, the patient's knee and hip are flexed and the examiner then adducts the leg to the contralateral hip. While executing this maneuver, the examiner presses on the knee to exert axial pressure on the femur.

b) To evaluate the sacrospinous and sacroiliac ligaments, the patient's knee and hip are maximally flexed and the examiner adducts the leg toward the contralateral shoulder. While executing this maneuver, the examiner presses on the knee to exert axial pressure on the femur.

c) To evaluate the sacrotuberal ligament, the patient's knee and hip are maximally flexed and the examiner moves the leg toward the ipsilateral shoulder.

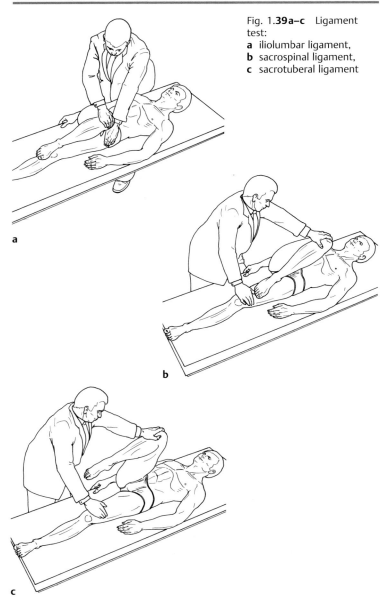

Fig. 1.**39a–c**   Ligament test:
**a** iliolumbar ligament,
**b** sacrospinal ligament,
**c** sacrotuberal ligament

**Assessment:** Stretching pain occurring within a few seconds suggests functional shortening and excessive stresses on the ligaments, although it can also occur in a hypermobile or motion-restricted sacroiliac joint.

Pain caused by stretching the iliolumbar ligament is referred to the inguinal region (the differential diagnosis includes a hip disorder). Pain caused by stretching the sacrospinous and sacroiliac ligaments is felt within the S1 dermatome from a point posterolateral to the hip as far as the knee. Sacrotuberal ligament pain radiates into the posterior aspect of the thigh.

### Springing Test 1

Assesses facet hypermobility in the sacroiliac joint.

**Procedure:** The patient is prone. The examiner places the index finger of one hand first on the superior margin of the sacroiliac joint and then on its inferior margin (S1–S3) in such a manner that the fingertip lies on the sacrum and the volar aspect of the distal phalanx lies on the medial margin of the ilium.

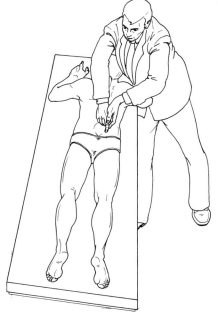

Fig. 1.**40**  Springing test

The examiner's other hand grasps the index finger and exerts posteroanterior pressure which the palpating finger transmits to the sacrum.

**Assessment:**   A normal sacroiliac joint will be resilient: palpating pressure will slightly increase the distance between the posterior margin of the ilium and the sacrum. This resiliency is not present in a motion-restricted sacroiliac joint. A relatively long range of motion with a hard endpoint suggests hypermobility in the sacroiliac joint. Pain during the examination can occur in both a motion-restricted and a strained hypermobile joint (painful hypermobility).

### Patrick Test (Fabere Sign)

Differentiates hip disorders from disorders of the sacroiliac joints (assessment of adductor tension).

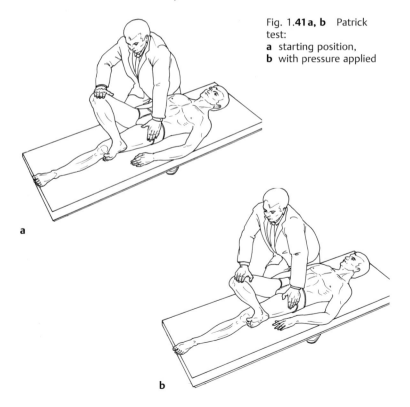

Fig. 1.**41a, b**   Patrick test:
**a** starting position,
**b** with pressure applied

a

b

**Procedure:** The patient is supine with one leg extended and the other flexed at the knee. The lateral malleolus of the flexed leg lies across the other leg superior to the patella.

The test may also be performed so that the foot of the flexed leg is in contact with the medial aspect of the knee of the contralateral leg. The flexed leg is then pressed or allowed to fall further into abduction. The examiner must immobilize the pelvis on the extended contralateral side to prevent it from moving during the test.

**Assessment:** Normally the knee of the abducted leg will almost touch the examining table. Comparative measurements of the distance between the knee and the table on both sides are made. A difference in mobility with painfully restricted motion in hyperabduction suggests the absence of a hip disorder; normal adductors suggest dysfunction in the ipsilateral sacroiliac joint. Hip disorders are excluded by testing range of motion in the hip (especially rotation) and palpating the hip capsule deep in the groin.

### Three-Phase Hyperextension Test

**Procedure:** The patient is prone. In the first phase of the test, the examiner grasps the patient's extended leg and raises it into hyperextension while immobilizing the pelvis with the other hand.

In the second phase, the examiner immobilizes the patient's sacrum parallel to the sacroiliac joint with the same hand and passively raises the patient's leg into hyperextension. In the third phase, the examiner immobilizes the fifth lumbar vertebra with the heel of one hand while passively guiding the patient's leg into hyperextension with the other hand. By moving the immobilizing hand up the spine, the examiner also evaluate higher segments of the lumbar spine.

**Assessment:** Under normal conditions no pain should occur in any phase of the test. The hip should allow about 10°–20° of hyperextension. The sacroiliac joint should exhibit slight play, and the lumbar spine should allow elastic hyperextension (lordosis) at the lumbosacral junction.

Pain with the ilium immobilized (phase 1) suggests a hip disorder or muscle contracture (rectus femoris and/or psoas). Pain when the sacrum is immobilized suggests motion restriction of the sacroiliac joint or other disorders of this joint, such as ankylosing spondylitis, while pain when the lumbar spine is immobilized suggests a disorder of the lumbosacral junction (vertebral motion restriction or protrusion or extrusion of an intervertebral disk).

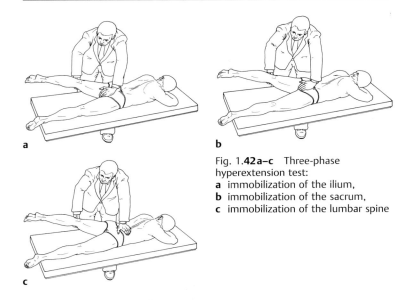

**a**

**b**

Fig. 1.**42a–c**  Three-phase
hyperextension test:
**a** immobilization of the ilium,
**b** immobilization of the sacrum,
**c** immobilization of the lumbar spine

**c**

**Note:**  The test for a Mennell sign is identical to the second phase of the three-phase hyperextension test.

## Spine Test

Assesses sacroiliac joint function.

**Procedure:**  The examiner stands behind the standing patient and palpates the posterior superior iliac spine and the median sacral crest (spinous processes of the fused sacral vertebrae) at the same level. The patient is asked to raise the ipsilateral leg and push his or her knee as far forward as possible.

**Assessment:**  If the sacroiliac joint is not motion-restricted, the ilium will move downward on the side being examined. The posterior superior iliac spine will be seen to shift inferiorly about 0.5 cm or up to at most 2 cm with the movement. This downward shift will not occur if the sacroiliac joint is motion-restricted; in fact, the motion restriction will usually cause the posterior superior iliac spine to move upwards (superiorly) as the pelvis tilts in compensation.

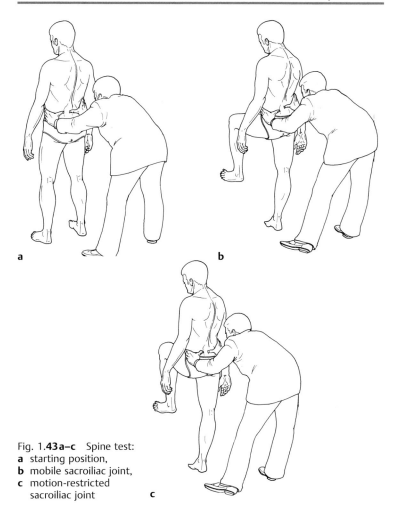

Fig. 1.**43a–c** Spine test:
**a** starting position,
**b** mobile sacroiliac joint,
**c** motion-restricted
sacroiliac joint

## Standing Flexion Test

Assesses sacroiliac joint function.

**Procedure:** The patient stands with his or her back to the examiner. The examiner's thumbs simultaneously palpate both posterior superior iliac spines. The patient is asked to slowly bend over while keeping both feet in contact with the floor and the knees extended. The examiner observes the position and/or motion of both iliac spines as the patient's torso bends forward.

**Assessment:**   The sacrum rotates relative to the ilia around a horizontal axis in the sacroiliac joints. This motion is referred to as "nutation."

In normal patients with mobile sacroiliac joints, both posterior superior iliac spines will be level with each other throughout the range of motion when the patient bends over.

If nutation does not occur in the sacroiliac joint on one side, the posterior superior iliac spine on that side will come to rest farther superior with respect to the sacrum than the spine on the contralateral side.

Where nutation fails to occur or this relative superior advancement is observed, this is usually a sign of a blockade in the ipsilateral sacroiliac joint. Bilateral superior advancement can be simulated by bilateral shortening of the hamstrings.

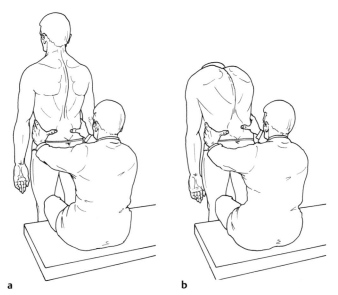

**a**                                          **b**

Fig. 1.**44a, b**   Standing flexion test:
**a** starting position,
**b** motion-restricted right sacroiliac joint

**Note:** When evaluating this superior advancement phenomenon, the examiner must consider or exclude possible asymmetry of the pelvis and hips. Pelvic obliquity due to a difference in leg length should be compensated for by placing shims under the shorter leg.

The standing flexion test can also be performed with the patient supine. The supine patient is asked to sit up (the patient may use his or her arms for support on the edge of the examining table). The examiner places both thumbs on the tips of the medial malleoli. As the patient sits up, the right malleolus will be seen to "advance" asymmetrically compared with its position in the supine patient. This is a sign of impaired mobility in the right sacroiliac joints.

### Sacroiliac Mobilization Test

Assesses sacroiliac joint function.

**Procedure:** The patient is prone. The examiner places the fingers of the palpating hand over the sacroiliac joints, i.e., over the posterior sacral ligaments (the sacroiliac joint itself is not accessible to palpation because of its anatomic position). The examiner places the other hand around the anterior iliac wing. With this hand, the examiner performs

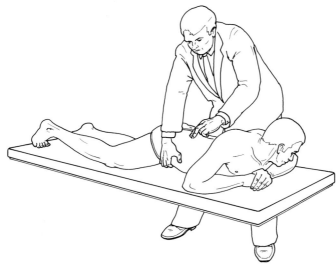

Fig. 1.**45**   Sacroiliac mobilization test

small shaking and lifting motions in a posterior direction (moving the ilium posteriorly relative to the sacrum).

**Assessment:** The palpating fingers over the sacroiliac joint will detect resilient motion in a normal joint, or painfully limited resiliency in the presence of a blockade.

### Sacroiliac Joint Springing Test 2

**Procedure:** To directly test the play in the sacroiliac joint, the patient is placed supine. The leg opposite the examiner is flexed at the knee and hip and adducted toward the examiner until the pelvis begins to follow. The other leg remains extended. Next, the examiner grasps the knee of the adducted leg and palpates the sacroiliac joint with the other hand while exerting resilient axial pressure on the knee.

**Assessment:** This maneuver normally produces a springy motion in the sacroiliac joint, which will be palpable as movement between the posterior iliac spine and the sacrum. Lack of joint play is typical of a functional impairment. This spring test is based on the knowledge that the range of motion in an intact joint can be increased by resilient pressure even with the joint at the extreme end of its range of motion. This essentially allows the diagnosis of a functional impairment in any joint by manual manipulation. However, the important thing is to perform the test with initial stress already applied to the joint. This test is recommended to supplement the prone spring tests.

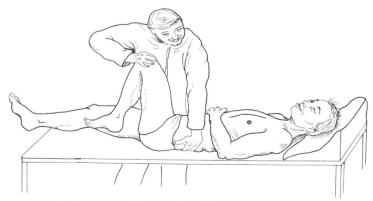

Fig. 1.**46**   Springing test of the sacroiliac joint

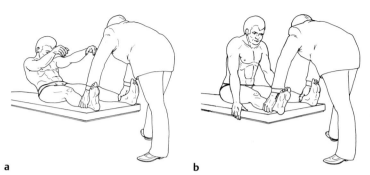

**a**                                                      **b**

Fig. 1.**47 a, b**  Derbolowsky sign:
**a**  mobile sacroiliac joint,
**b**  motion-restricted right sacroiliac joint (causes leg lengthening when the patient sits up)

## Derbolowsky Sign

Assesses a leg length difference: an advancement phenomenon with the patient supine.

**Procedure:**  The patient is supine. The examiner grasps both ankles, palpates the patient's medial malleoli with each thumb, and evaluates the relative level and rotation of the medial malleoli.

The patient is asked to sit up. The examiner may either help the patient do so, or the patient may use his or her hands for support.

**Assessment:**  Where there is a motion restriction in the sacroiliac joint without any play between the sacrum and ilium, the ipsilateral leg will be longer when the patient sits up and apparently shorter or the same length as the other leg when the patient is supine. The examiner measures the difference in the level of the two malleoli, which previously were at the same level. A difference of less than 2 cm is not significant. The differential diagnosis should consider whether something other than a motion restriction in the sacroiliac joint may be causing the variable leg length difference. Possible such causes include shortening of the hamstrings or genuine anatomic leg lengthening or shortening.

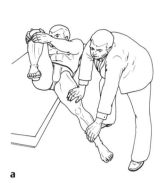 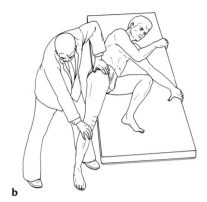

Fig. 1.**48a, b**   Gaenslen sign:
**a** supine,
**b** lateral position

## Gaenslen Sign (2nd Mennell Sign)

Assesses sacroiliac joint function.

**Procedure:**   The patient is supine with the painful side as close as possible to the edge of the examining table or projecting beyond it. To stabilize this position and immobilize the lumbar spine, the patient flexes the knee and hip of the contralateral leg and draws the leg as close to the torso as possible (Thomas grip). The examiner then passively hyperextends the leg next to the edge of the examining table.

The test may also be performed with the patient in a lateral position. This is done with the patient lying on his or her normal side with that leg flexed at the hip and knee. The examiner then passively hyperextends the other leg (the one not in contact with the table).

• **Assessment:**   If there is dysfunction in the sacroiliac joint, hyperextension of the leg will lead to motion in the sacroiliac joint, causing pain or exacerbation of existing pain.

Pain may also be caused by hip pathology or an ipsilateral nerve root lesion.

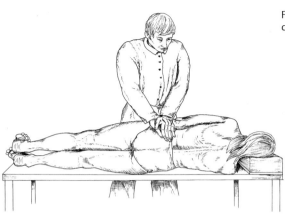

Fig. 1.**49**  Iliac compression test

## Iliac Compression Test

Indicates sacroiliac disease.

**Procedure:**  The patient is a lateral position. The examiner places both hands on the ilium of the affected side and exerts downward pressure on the pelvis.

**Assessment:**  Occurrence of or an increase in pain in the sacroiliac joint adjacent to the examiner's hand suggests a joint disorder (such as motion restriction or inflammation).

## 1st Mennell Sign

Indicates sacroiliac disease.

**Procedure:**  The patient is prone. When examining the left sacroiliac joint, the examiner immobilizes the patient's sacrum with the left hand while grasping the patient's extended left leg with the right hand and suddenly hyperextending the hip.

The examination may also be performed with the patient in a lateral position. This is done with patient lying on his or her right side and immobilizing that leg, flexed at the hip and knee, with both hands. The examiner stands behind the patient holding the patient's pelvis with his or her right hand and then suddenly hyperextends the patient's left hip with the left hand.

**Assessment:**  Pain in the sacroiliac joint suggests a joint disorder (such as motion restriction or inflammation).

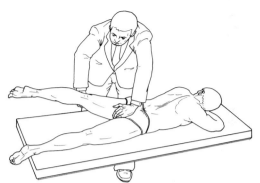

Fig. 1.**50**   Mennell sign

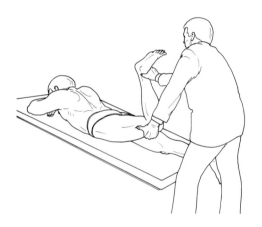

Fig. 1.**51**   Yeoman test

## Yeoman Test

Assesses sacroiliac pain.

**Procedure:**   The patient is prone with the knee flexed 90°. The examiner raises the flexed leg off the examining table, hyperextending the hip.

**Assessment:**   The first part of this test initially places stress on the posterior structures of the sacroiliac joint; later the stress shifts to the anterior portions, primarily affecting the anterior sacroiliac ligaments. Pain in the lumbar spine suggests the presence of pathologic processes at that site. Anterior thigh paresthesia may indicate a femoral nerve stretch.

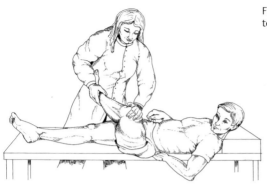

Fig. 1.**52**  Laguerre test

## Laguerre Test

Differentiates hip pain from sacroiliac pain.

**Procedure:**  The patient is supine. The examiner passively flexes the patient's hip and knee 90°. Then the hip is passively abducted and placed in extreme external rotation.

**Assessment:**  This maneuver moves the femoral head into the anterior part of the joint capsule of the hip. Pain within the hip suggests degenerative joint disease, hip dysplasia, or contracture of the iliopsoas. Pain felt posteriorly in the sacroiliac joint suggests a disease process at that site.

## Sacroiliac Stress Test

Demonstrates involvement of the anterior sacroiliac ligaments in a sacroiliac joint syndrome.

**Procedure:**  The patient is supine. The examiner exerts anterior pressure on the iliac wings with both hands. By crossing his or her hands, the examiner adds a lateral force vector to the compression. The anteroposterior direction of the compressive load on the pelvis places stress on the posterior portions of the sacroiliac joint, whereas the lateral component places stress on the anterior sacroiliac ligaments.

**Assessment:**  Deep pain is a sign of strained anterior sacroiliac ligaments on the side of the pain (sacrospinal and sacrotuberal ligaments). Pain in the buttocks can be produced by compression from the examining table or by irritation of the posterior portions of the sacroiliac joint. Determining the precise location of the pain helps to identify its cause.

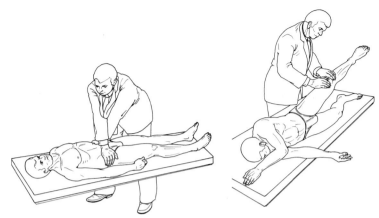

Fig. 1.**53**   Sacroiliac stress test          Fig. 1.**54**   Abduction stress test

### Abduction Stress Test

Indicates a sacroiliac joint syndrome.

**Procedure:**   The patient is in a lateral position. With the leg in contact with the table flexed, the patient attempts to continue to abduct the upper extended leg against the examiner's resistance. This test is normally performed to evaluate insufficiency of the gluteus medius and gluteus minimus.

**Assessment:**   Increasing pain in the affected sacroiliac joint is a sign of sacroiliac irritation. Patients with hip disorders may also feel increased pain when this test is performed. The location of the pain is suggestive of the type of disorder. A leg that can only be abducted slightly or not at all without causing pain suggests insufficiency of the gluteus minimus.

## ■ Nerve Root Compression Syndrome

Disk extrusions usually lead to nerve compression syndromes with radicular pain. The pain in the sacrum and leg is often exacerbated by coughing, sneezing, pushing, or even simply walking. Mobility in the spine is severely limited by pain, and there is significant tension in the lumbar musculature. Sensory and motor deficits and impaired reflexes are additional symptoms that occur with nerve root compression.

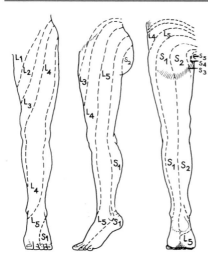

Fig. 1.**55** Dermatomes of the lumbar and sacral plexuses according to Herlin. The L4 dermatome rarely extends as far as the foot, and the sole of the foot is rarely supplied in part by the posterior L5 root

Often the affected nerve root can be identified by the description of the paresthesia and radiating pain in the dermatome. Extrusions of the fourth and fifth lumbar disks are especially common, extrusions of the third lumbar disk less so. Disk extrusions involving the first and second lumbar disks are rare.

The Lasègue sign is usually positive (often even at 20°–30°) in compression of the L5–S1 nerve root (typical sciatica). In these cases, even passively raising the normal leg will often elicit or exacerbate pain in the lower back and the affected leg (contralateral Lasègue sign). In nerve root compression syndromes from L1 through L4 with involvement of the femoral nerve, the Lasègue sign is rarely positive and then only slightly and only when the L4 nerve root is affected.

When the femoral nerve is irritated, the reverse Lasègue sign and/or pain from stretching of the femoral nerve can usually be triggered.

Pseudo-radicular pain must be distinguished from genuine radicular pain (sciatica). Pseudo-radicular pain is usually less circumscribed than radicular pain. Facet syndrome (arthritis in the facet joints), sacroiliac joint syndrome, painful spondylolisthesis, stenosis of the spinal canal, and postdiskectomy syndrome are clinical pictures that frequently cause pseudo-radicular pain.

Table 1.**3**   Signs of radicular symptoms

| Root | Dermatome Pain | Sensory deficit | Paralyzed muscles | Impaired reflexes |
|------|----------------|-----------------|-------------------|-------------------|
| L2 L1–L2 Extraforaminal: L2-L3 | Thoracolumbar junction, sacroiliac joint, groin, iliac crest, proximal medial thigh | Groin, proximal anterior and medial thigh | Paresis of the iliopsoas, quadriceps femoris, and adductors (slight) | Cremaster and patellar reflex weakened |
| L3 L2–L3 Extraforaminal: L3-L4 | Upper lumbar spine, anterior proximal thigh | From the anterior thigh to the medial thigh and distal to the knee | Paresis of the iliopsoas, quadriceps femoris, and adductors (slight) | Absent or weakened patellar reflex |
| L4 L2–L3 Extraforaminal: L3-L4 | Lumbar spine, anterolateral thigh, hip region | From the lateral thigh to the medial lower leg and margin of the foot | Paresis of the quadriceps femoris and tibialis anterior (difficulty walking on heels) | Weakened patellar reflex |
| L5 L4–L5 Extraforaminal: L5-S1 | Lumbar spine, posterior thigh, lateral lower leg, medial foot, groin, hip region | From the lateral lower leg to the medial foot (great toe) | Paresis of the extensor hallucis longus and brevis, extensor digitorum longus and brevis (difficulty walking on heels) | Loss of tibialis posterior reflex (significant only when readily elicited on contralateral side) |
| S1 L5–S1 | Lumbar spine, posterior thigh, posterolateral lower leg, lateral margin of foot, sole of foot, groin, hip region, coccyx | Posterior aspect of the thigh and lower leg, lateral margin of the foot and sole of the foot (little toe) | Paresis of the peroneus muscles and triceps surae (difficulty walking on tiptoes; foot bends laterally) | Weakening or loss of Achilles tendon reflex |

## Slump Test

**Procedure:** The patient is seated on the edge of the examining table with the legs supported. The hips are in a neutral position and the hands are placed behind the back. The examination is performed step by step.

First the patient is asked to "slump" the back into thoracic and lumbar flexion. The head is kept in a neutral position, which is provided by the examiner holding the patient's chin. The examiner then applies pressure across the shoulders with the other arm to maintain flexion in the thoracic and lumbar spine. The patient is then asked to actively flex the cervical spine and head as far as possible in this position. The examiner then applies pressure to maintain flexion in all three parts

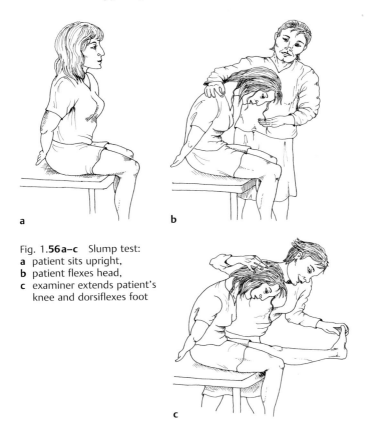

Fig. 1.**56a–c** Slump test:
**a** patient sits upright,
**b** patient flexes head,
**c** examiner extends patient's knee and dorsiflexes foot

of the spine. The hand of the same arm is used. With the other hand the examiner holds the patient's foot in maximum dorsiflexion. In this position the patient is asked to actively straighten the knee as much as possible.

The test is repeated with the other leg and then with both legs at the same time.

**Assessment:**  The test can cause impingement of the dura, spinal cord, or nerve roots with pain radiating down into the areas supplied by the sciatic nerve.

The test also places stress on other tissues. Some discomfort or pain is not necessarily pathognomonic.

Nonpathological response includes pain or discomfort in the region T8–T9, pain or discomfort of the hamstrings behind the extended knee, symmetric restriction of the knee extension, symmetric restriction of ankle dorsiflexion, and increased symmetric knee extension and ankle dorsiflexion on release of neck flexion.

### Lasègue Sign (Straight Leg Raising Test)

Indicates nerve root irritation.

**Procedure:**  The examiner slowly raises the patient's leg (extended at the knee) until the patient reports pain.

**Assessment:**  Intense pain in the sacrum and leg suggests nerve root irritation (disk extrusion or tumor). However, a genuine positive Lasègue sign is only present where the pain shoots into the leg explo-

Fig. 1.**57**  Lasègue sign

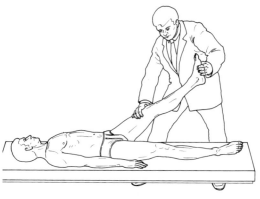

sively along a course corresponding to the motor and sensory derma-tome of the affected nerve root.

The patient often attempts to avoid the pain by lifting the pelvis on the side being examined.

The angle achieved when lifting the leg is estimated in degrees. This angle gives an indication of severity of the nerve root irritation present (genuine Lasègue Sign is at 60° or less).

Sciatica can also be provoked by adducting and internally rotating the leg with the knee flexed. This test is also described as a Bonnet or piriformis sign (adduction and internal rotation of the leg stretches the nerve as it passes through the piriformis).

Increases in sciatica pain by raising the head (Kernig sign) and/or passive dorsiflexion of the great toes (Turyn sign) are further signs of significant sciatic nerve irritation (differential diagnosis should consider meningitis, subarachnoid hemorrhage, and carcinomatous meningitis).

Sacral or lumbar pain that increases only slowly as the leg is raised or pain radiating into the posterior thigh is usually attributable to degen-erative joint disease (facet syndrome), irritation of the pelvic ligaments (tendinitis), or increased tension or shortening in the hamstrings (in-dicated by a soft endpoint, usually also found on the contralateral side). It is important to distinguish this "pseudo-radicular" pain (pseudo-Lasègue sign) from genuine sciatica (true Lasègue sign).

Normally the leg can be raised 15°–30° before the nerve root is stretched in the intervertebral foramen. Pain occurring at over 60° of flexion suggests joint pain in the lumbar area (e.g., facet joints or sacroiliac joints). It is important to compare both in order to decide whether pain is caused by stretching of the neurologic tissue or arises from the joints or other soft tissues.

If one leg is lifted and pain occurs on the opposite side this can indicate a space-occupying lesion such as a herniated disk or an inflam-matory swelling. This may be called the crossover sign and usually indicates a rather large medial intervertebral disk protrusion. The test causes stretching of the ipsilateral as well as the contralateral nerve root, pulling laterally on the dural sac. A positive Lasègue and crossover sign can also give an indication of the degree of disk injury. Many patients with a central protrusion are candidates for surgery, especially if there are bowel and bladder symptoms. For patients who have diffi-culty lying supine a modified straight leg raising test has been sug-gested.

The patient is in a lateral position with the test leg uppermost and the hip and knee in flexion of 90°. The lumbosacral spine normally is in a neutral position, but may be slightly flexed or extended as the patient's condition allows. The examiner then passively extends the patient's knee. Pain resistance and reproduction of the patient's symptoms indicate a positive test.

It can also be impossible to lift the leg at the hip if the patient consciously resists this and attempts to press the leg downward against the examiner's hand. Occasionally one will encounter this behavior in experienced patients undergoing examination within the scope of an expert opinion (see Lasègue test with the patient seated).

### Bonnet Sign (Piriformis Sign)

**Procedure:**   The patient is supine with the leg flexed at the hip and knee. The examiner adducts and internally rotates the leg.

**Assessment:**   The Lasègue sign occurs earlier in this maneuver. The nerve is stretched as it passes through the piriformis, resulting in increased pain.

### Lasègue Test with the Patient Seated

Indicates nerve root irritation.

**Procedure:**   The patient sits on the edge of the examining table and is asked to flex his or her hip with the leg extended at the knee.

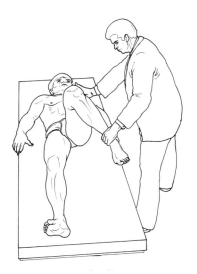

Fig. 1.**58**   Bonnet sign

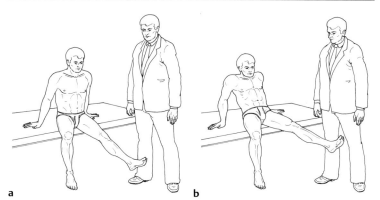

Fig. 1.**59a, b** Lasègue sign with the patient seated:
**a** beginning hip flexion,
**b** with increasing hip flexion

**Assessment:** This test corresponds to the Lasègue sign. When nerve root irritation is present, the patient will avoid the pain by leaning backward and using his or her arms for support. This test can also be used to identify simulated pain. If the patient can readily flex the hip without leaning backward, then a previous positive Lasègue sign must be questioned. The examiner can also perform this test in the same manner as the test for the Lasègue sign by passively flexing the hip with the knee extended.

### Bragard Test

Indicates nerve root compression syndrome, differentiating a genuine Lasègue sign from a pseudo-Lasègue sign.

**Procedure:** The patient is supine. The examiner grasps the patient's heel with one hand and anterior aspect of the knee with the other. The examiner slowly raises the patient's leg, which is extended at the knee. At the onset of the Lasègue sign, the examiner lowers the patient's leg just far enough that the patient no longer feels pain. The examiner then passively moves the patient's foot into extreme dorsiflexion in this position, eliciting the typical pain caused by stretching of the sciatic nerve.

**Assessment:** A positive Bragard sign is evidence of nerve root compression, which may lie between L4 and S1.

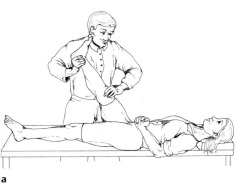

Fig. 1.**60a, b**    Bragard test:
**a** starting position,
**b** dorsiflexion of the foot

**a**

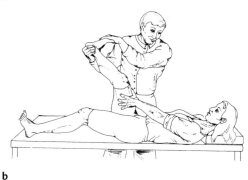

**b**

Dull, nonspecific pain in the posterior thigh radiating into the knee is attributable to stretching of the hamstrings and should not be assessed as a Lasègue sign.

A sensation of tension in the calf may be attributable to thrombosis, thrombophlebitis, or contracture of the gastrocnemius.

The Bragard sign can be used to test whether the patient is malingering. The sign is usually negative in malingerers.

### Lasègue Differential Test

Differentiates sciatica from a hip disorder.

**Procedure:**   The patient is supine. The examiner grasps the patient's heel with one hand and the anterior aspect of the knee with the other. The examiner slowly raises the patient's leg, which is extended at the

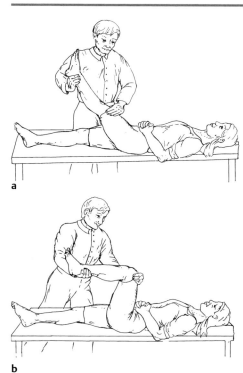

Fig. 1.**61a, b** Lasègue differential test:
**a** starting position,
**b** knee flexed

**a**

**b**

knee, until the patient feels pain. The examiner then notes the location and nature of the pain and estimates in degrees the maximum pain-free angle that can be achieved when lifting the leg.

The test is repeated and the leg is then flexed once the painful angle is reached.

**Assessment:** In a patient with sciatic nerve irritation, flexing the knee will significantly reduce symptoms, even to the point that they disappear completely. Where a hip disorder is present, the pain will remain and may even be exacerbated by increasing flexion in the hip.

**Note:** Pain in hip disorders is usually located in the groin and only rarely in the posterolateral region of the hip. Only in the case of posterolateral pain may it be hard to differentiate between nerve root irritation and pain caused by a hip disorder.

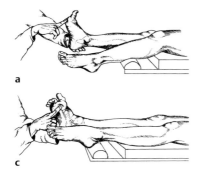

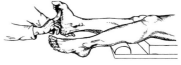

Fig. 1.**62a–c**　Duchenne sign:
**a** starting position,
**b** normal,
**c** abnormal

## Duchenne Sign

Assesses a nerve root disorder.

**Procedure:** The patient is supine. The examiner grasps the patient's heel with one hand and with one finger of the other hand presses the first metatarsal head posteriorly. From this position, the patient is asked to flex the foot.

**Assessment:** In the presence of a disk disorder involving the S1 nerve root, the patient will be unable to resist the finger pressure. Paresis of the peroneus muscles causes supination of the foot due to the action of the anterior and posterior tibial muscles.

## Kernig-Brudzinski Test

Indicates nerve root irritation.

**Procedure:** The patient is supine and is asked to flex the hip and knee of one leg. In the first part of the test, the examiner attempts to passively extend the patient's knee; in the second part, the patient actively attempts to flex the knee.

**Assessment:** Pain in the spine or radicular pain in the leg occurring during active or passive knee flexion suggests meningeal irritation, nerve root involvement, or dural irritation.

　　In the absence of pain during the active straight leg raise, the examiner may further elongate the spinal cord and increase the tension to the dural sheath by flexing the cervical spine passively—Brudzinski's portion of the test.

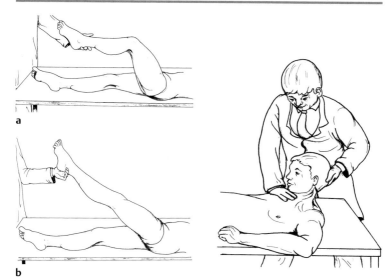

Fig. 1.**63a, b** Kernig test:
**a** starting position,
**b** knee flexed

Fig. **1.63c** Brudzinski sign

## Tiptoe and Heel Walking Test

Identifies and assesses a nerve root disorder in the lumbar spine.

**Procedure:** The patient is asked to stand first on his or her heels, then on tiptoe, and then to take a few steps in each of these positions if possible.

**Assessment:** Difficulty or inability to stand or walk on tiptoe suggests a lesion of the S1 nerve root; difficulty or inability to stand or walk on the heels suggests a lesion of the L4–L5 nerve root.

**Note:** A differential diagnosis must exclude a ruptured Achilles tendon. This injury makes it impossible to stand on tiptoe, especially when standing only on the affected leg.

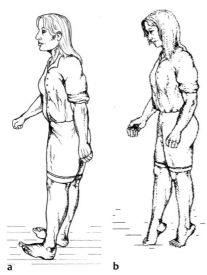

Fig. 1.**64a, b**   Tiptoe and heel walking test:
**a**   heel walking,
**b**   tiptoe walking

## Femoral Nerve Traction Test

**Procedure:**   The patient lies on the unaffected side with the unaffected limb flexed slightly at the hip and knee. The examiner grasps the patient's affected or painful limb and extends the knee while gently extending the hip. The patient's knee is then flexed.

**Assessment:**   Neurologic pain radiates down the anterior thigh if the test is positive.

This also is a traction test for the nerve roots of the midlumbar spine (L2–L4). As with the straight leg raising test, the contralateral test can also be positive when symptoms occur in the opposite lower limp. This is called the crossed femoral stretching test. Pain in the groin and hip radiating along the anterior medial thigh indicates an L3 nerve root problem; pain extending to the mid-tibia indicates an L4 nerve root problem.

The test is similar to the Ober test for a tight iliotibial band, so the examiner must be able to differentiate between the two conditions.

If the iliotibial band is tight, the leg being examined does not adduct but remains elevated away from the table as the tight tendon riding over the greater trochanter keeps the leg abducted.

Femoral nerve injury presents with a different history and the referred pain (anteriorly) tends to be stronger.

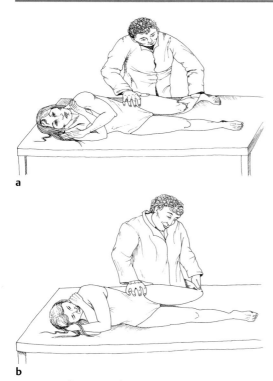

Fig. 1.**65a, b**  Femoral nerve traction test:
**a** extension of the hip; knee slightly flexed,
**b** flexion of the knee

### Reverse Lasègue Test (Femoral Nerve Lasègue Test)

Indicates nerve root irritation.

**Procedure:**  The patient is prone. The examiner passively raises the leg, which is flexed at the knee.

**Assessment:**  Hyperextension of the hip with the knee flexed places traction on the femoral nerve. Occurrence of unilateral or bilateral radicular pain in the sacrum or anterior thigh, rarely in the lower leg as well, is a sign of nerve root irritation. Pain in the groin and hip that radiates along the anterior medial thigh, indicates an L3 nerve root problem. Pain extending to the midtibia indicates an L4 nerve root

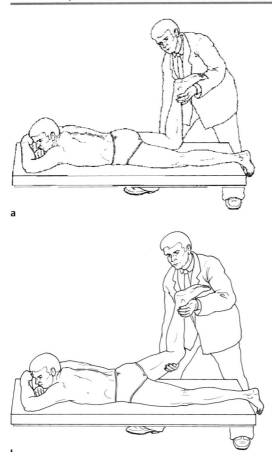

a

b

Fig. 1.**66a, b**   Reverse Lasègue test:
**a**  starting position,
**b**  hip hyperextended

problem. This should be differentiated from complaints caused by de-generative hip disease or by shortening of the rectus femoris or psoas.

**Note:**  With upper lumbar disk disturbance there may be weakness of the quadriceps muscle and a diminished or absent patellar reflex.

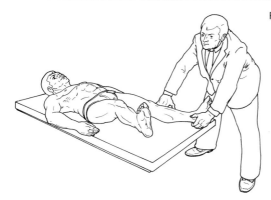

Fig. 1.**67** Hoover test

## Hoover Test

Evaluation of malingering.

**Procedure:** The patient lies supine. The examiner places one hand under each calcaneus. The patient is then asked to perform active straight leg raising. The knee is kept straight and the leg is actively lifted off the table.

**Assessment:** If the patient does not lift the leg or the examiner does not feel pressure under the opposite heel, the patient is probably not really trying or may be a malingerer. If the lifted limb is weaker, pressure under the normal heel increases, because of the increased effort to lift the weak leg off the examination table. Often patients will report that they cannot raise the leg at all. Both sides have to be compared for differences.

# 2 Shoulder

Acute injuries and chronic complaints in the shoulder have become increasingly important in recent years. Contributing factors include occupational, recreational, and sports activities. Years of occupational, recreational, or household activities involving overhead work lead to excessive stresses and muscle imbalance as does sitting at an unergonomic workplace like many secretaries.

As in any clinical examination, the first step in examining the shoulder is to obtain a thorough history. The many different shoulder disorders may have their causes in acute trauma, local processes due to chronic overuse, age-related degeneration, or systemic disease. In adolescence and early adulthood, shoulder disorders are primarily attributable to trauma or congenital deformities. The most common of these shoulder disorders include dislocations and subluxations and their resulting instabilities. Later in life, degenerative disorders become more prominent. These include impingement syndrome, ruptures of the rotator cuff, and degenerative acromioclavicular joint changes.

Inquiring about occupational stresses and athletic activities provides important information. Jobs involving a lot of overhead work (painting) and sports with similar requirements (basketball, baseball, tennis, swimming, volleyball) often lead to early disorders in the subacromial space. These are accompanied by degenerative changes in the acromioclavicular joint. Obtaining a detailed history from an athlete requires knowledge of the motion sequences specific to his or her respective sport. This is crucial to diagnosing patterns of injury specific to that sport.

However, acute symptoms are not always attributable to obvious trauma from an identifiable mechanism of injury. In the presence of preexisting tendon degeneration, a minor injury can lead to a supraspinatus tendon rupture.

In addition to specific questions about shoulder disorders, the examiner must always be alert to the possibility of diseases of other organ systems. Pain from angina pectoris often radiates into the shoulder and arm, and this referred pain does not invariably occur on the left side. Gallbladder or liver disorders can also cause pain in the right shoulder. Rheumatic polyarthritis and hyperuricemia can manifest first in the shoulder. Patients with diabetes mellitus very often have an associated shoulder affliction that tends to restrict motion in the shoulder. One of the most common neoplastic causes of shoulder pain is a Pancoast tumor with a typical Horner syndrome.

Observing the patient provides the examiner with an initial overview. Gait and any compensatory contralateral motion of the upper extremities are noted. A patient with a frozen shoulder avoids internal or external rotation and motion above horizontal when undressing. Patients with a ruptured rotator cuff will often ask for help undressing because they lack the strength to abduct the arm. Asymmetry and especially muscle atrophy is best revealed by comparison with the contralateral side. In comparative inspection of both acromioclavicular joints, the examiner looks for swelling or a step off resulting from an acromioclavicular joint separation. Distal displacement of the muscle belly suggests a rupture of the long head of the biceps tendon. The same applies to many congenital disorders such as a Sprengel deformity, Klippel–Feil syndrome, congenital torticollis, or the clavicular fracture often seen in newborns and infants. Isolated supraspinatus atrophy suggests a rupture of this tendon.

Distal compression neuropathies and thoracic outlet syndrome also first manifest themselves as shoulder pain.

AP and lateral radiographs and special shoulder views are indicated to supplement the clinical examination. These can differentiate bony changes from soft tissue pathology. Ultrasound, MRI, and CT may also be useful in visualizing shoulder disorders.

# Range of Motion of the Shoulder (Neutral-Zero Method)

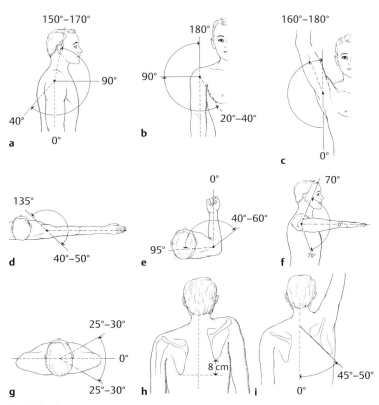

Fig. **2.1 a–i**

**a**  Forward flexion and extension.

**b**  Abduction and adduction.

**c**  Abduction exceeding 90° requires external rotation of the humerus in the glenohumeral joint and rotation of scapula.

**d**  Horizontal flexion and extension (forward and backward motion of the arm, abducted 90° from the body).

**e, f**  External and internal rotation: with the arm hanging down (**e**) and abducted 90° (**f**).

**g**  Protraction and retraction of the shoulder.

**h**  Scapular elevation and depression.

**i**  Scapular rotation relative to the trunk

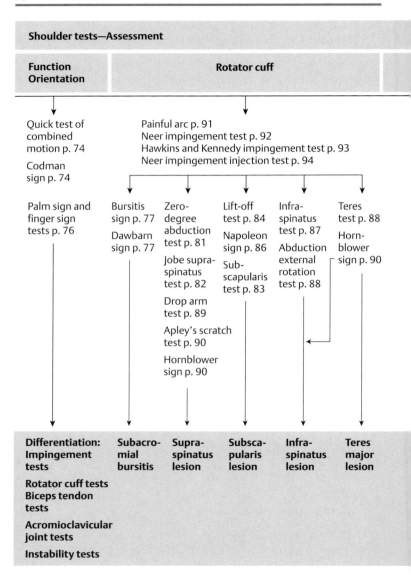

Fig. 2.**2**   Shoulder tests

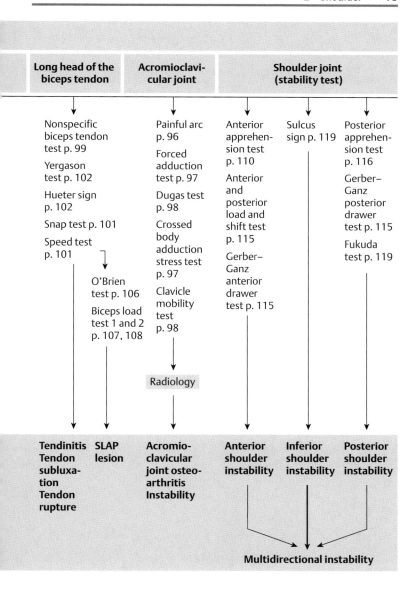

| Long head of the biceps tendon | Acromioclavicular joint | Shoulder joint (stability test) | | |
|---|---|---|---|---|

Nonspecific biceps tendon test p. 99

Yergason test p. 102

Hueter sign p. 102

Snap test p. 101

Speed test p. 101

O'Brien test p. 106

Biceps load test 1 and 2 p. 107, 108

Painful arc p. 96

Forced adduction test p. 97

Dugas test p. 98

Crossed body adduction stress test p. 97

Clavicle mobility test p. 98

Radiology

Anterior apprehension test p. 110

Anterior and posterior load and shift test p. 115

Gerber–Ganz anterior drawer test p. 115

Sulcus sign p. 119

Posterior apprehension test p. 116

Gerber–Ganz posterior drawer test p. 115

Fukuda test p. 119

**Tendinitis Tendon subluxation Tendon rupture**

**SLAP lesion**

**Acromioclavicular joint osteoarthritis Instability**

**Anterior shoulder instability**

**Inferior shoulder instability**

**Posterior shoulder instability**

**Multidirectional instability**

# ■ Orientation Tests

## Quick Test of Combined Motion

**Procedure:**   A quick test of mobility in the shoulder is to ask the patient to place hand behind his or her head and touch the contralateral scapula. In a second movement the patient places the hand behind his or her back, reaching upward from the buttocks to touch the inferior margin of the scapula.

**Assessment:**   Mobility on one side that is restricted in comparison with the contralateral side is a sign that a shoulder disorder exists. Other tests may then be used to diagnose this disorder in greater detail. Pain indicates degenerative tendinitis of one of the tendons of the rotator cuff, usually the supraspinatus tendon, or adhesive capsulitis.

## Codman Sign

Tests passive motion in the shoulder.

**Procedure:**   The examiner stands behind the patient and places his or her hand on the patient's shoulder so that the thumb immobilizes the patient's scapula slightly below the scapular spine, the index rests on

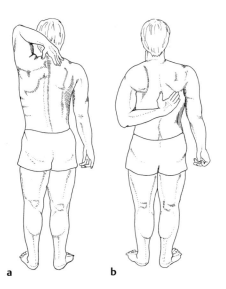

Fig. 2.**3a, b**   Quick test of combined motion:
**a** touching the scapula from behind the neck,
**b** touching the scapula from behind the back

a                          b

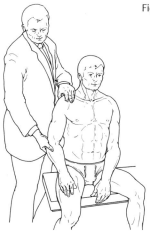

Fig. 2.**4**  Codman sign

the anterior margin of the acromion toward the tip of the coracoid, and the remaining fingers extend anteriorly past the acromion.

The examiner then moves the patient's arm in every direction using the other hand.

**Assessment:**  The examiner notes any crepitation in the glenohumeral joint, snapping phenomena (such as dislocations of the long head of the biceps tendon), or restricted motion.

The most important bony pressure points, such as the greater and lesser tubercles of the humerus, coracoid process, and sternoclavicular and acromioclavicular joints, are assessed for tenderness to palpation. Joint stability is also assessed, and pain in the tendons of the rotator cuff is evaluated by palpation.

The range of motion is determined using the neutral-zero method. The active and passive ranges of motion are determined, as are the region of occurrence and specific localization of symptoms. Restricted motion in every direction indicates the presence of a "frozen shoulder."

In the early stages of a rotator cuff tear, only active motion is restricted; passive motion remains normal. A chronic tear or advanced impingement syndrome will exhibit the universally restricted motion of a frozen shoulder.

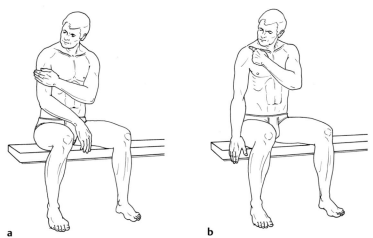

Fig. 2.**5a, b**    Palm sign test and finger sign test:
**a** palm sign,
**b** finger sign

## Palm Sign Test and Finger Sign Test

Typically, shoulder pain begins in the shoulder and radiates into the upper arm. Patients usually describe this pain in two ways. The "palm sign" is typical of glenohumeral and subacromial pain; the patient places the palm of the normal contralateral hand directly under the acromion.

The "palm sign" is typical of pain in the acromioclavicular joint; in this case, the patient places the finger of the normal contralateral hand directly on the affected acromioclavicular joint.

## ▪ Bursitis Tests

### Bursae

The shoulder contains a series of bursae. Communicating structures include the subscapular and subcoracoid bursae, and the subdeltoid bursa with its subacromial extension. They ensure smooth motion between the rotator cuff and acromion and acromioclavicular joint that lie superficial to it. They usually cause significant pain in shoulder pathology. These bursae often combine to form a synovial bursa.

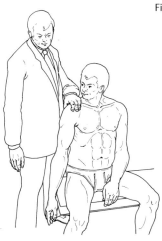

Fig. 2.**6**   Subacromial bursitis sign

## Bursitis Sign

Diagnosis of shoulder pains of uncertain etiology.

**Procedure:** The examiner palpates the anterolateral subacromial region with his or her index and middle fingers.

The examiner can expand the subacromial space by passively extending or hyperextending the patient's arm with the other hand and pressing the humeral head forward with the thumb. This also allows palpation of the superior portions of the rotator cuff and its insertions into the greater tubercle of the humerus.

**Assessment:**   Localized tenderness to palpation in the subacromial space suggests irritation of the subacromial bursa but can also be a sign of a rotator cuff disorder.

## Dawbarn Test

Sign of subacromial bursitis.

**Procedure:**   While further abducting the patient's moderately abducted arm with one hand, the examiner palpates the anterolateral subacromial space with the other hand.

The examiner exerts additional focal subacromial pressure while passively abducting the patient's arm up to 90°.

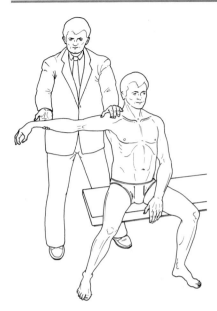

Fig. 2.**7**    Dawbarn test

**Assessment:**   Subacromial pain that decreases with abduction suggests bursitis, also a rotator cuff lesion. In abduction, the deltoid glides over the margin of the subacromial bursa, reducing the pain.

## ■ Rotator Cuff (Impingement Symptoms)

Pain and varying degrees of functional impairment are typically the dominant features in the clinical picture of a rotator cuff lesion.

In the phase of acute pain, it will usually be difficult to obtain sufficient information from the examination to determine whether the shoulder is due to calcification, tendinitis, subscapularis syndrome, or a rotator cuff tear. It is even more difficult to distinguish a rotator cuff tear from disorders caused by degenerative tendon changes without rupture. Clinical classification of shoulder pain and muscle weakness only becomes easier once the pain of the acute phase has abated.

Active motion is nearly normal, but reduced overall, in supraspinatus tears involving the anterior superior portion. The loss of active motion is more pronounced in injuries to the posterior portion and most extreme in complete tears. However, this is only an indication; the range of motion does not allow conclusions about the type of the lesion.

Pseudo-stiffening of the shoulder must be distinguished from "frozen shoulder." Pseudo-stiffening is often caused advanced but minimally painful osteoarthritis in the sternoclavicular joint. If this change is not considered, one risks mistakenly attributing the decreased range of motion to changes in the glenohumeral joint. A good test to distinguish these two is to watch the patient shrug (elevate the shoulders); a limited range of motion may only be attributed to glenohumeral joint pathology where elevation of the shoulders is normal.

Scapular and thoracic pathology must be excluded in the same manner. A "creaking" shoulder due to a bony projection such as scapular or costal osteophytes is less serious than the scapula that becomes fixed in a posterior thoracic defect, such as can occur secondary to thoracoplasty or multiple fractures of adjacent ribs. It is equally important to exclude dysfunction of the shoulder musculature, whether the scapular and thoracic or the glenohumeral musculature. The examiner should be particularly alert to the possibility of a serratus muscle palsy, which is tested for by verifying whether the scapula lifts off when pushing away the patient with his or her arms in forward extension. Paralysis of the trapezius must also be excluded. This paralysis limits mobility in the shoulder because the scapula can no longer be immobilized. The ability to elevate the scapula rules out this paralysis, as does the ability to elevate the shoulders (in shrugging).

Even under normal circumstances, there is little space available for the structures that lie beneath the coracoacromial arch. This space is further diminished when the greater tubercle of the humerus moves beneath the acromion in elevation. The supraspinatus is particularly affected by this confinement. The space available for its motion is limited on all sides by the anterior acromion, the coracoacromial ligament, the acromioclavicular joint, and the coracoid process (the supraspinatus outlet).

Impingement syndrome is a painful functional impairment of the shoulder that occurs when the rotator tendons impinge on the anterior margin of the coracoacromial arch and/or the acromioclavicular joint. The rotator cuff and the bursa beneath it can be locally compressed on the anterior margin of the acromion in elevation, and against the coracoid process in internal rotation. A subacromial or subcoracoid impingement syndrome can occur. Impingement lesions can also involve structures other than the rotator cuff that lie in the impingement zone, such as the biceps tendon and the subacromial bursa.

According to Neer, a distinction is made between primary impingement (outlet impingement) and secondary impingement (nonoutlet impingement). Primary impingement involves irritation of the supraspinatus as a result of mechanical constriction (in the supraspinatus outlet). Contributing factors may include congenital changes in the shape of the acromion, acquired bone spurs on the anterior margin of the acromion, inferior osteophytes on the acromioclavicular joint, and posttraumatic deformities of the coracoid process, acromion, and greater tubercle of the humerus. Secondary impingement (subacromial syndrome) involves relative constriction of the subacromial space due to the increase in volume of the structures that pass beneath the coracoacromial arch. Thickening of the rotator cuff and bursa (due to calcifications or chronic bursitis) and posttraumatic superior displacement of the greater tubercle of the humerus are the most common causes.

The failure of the depressor muscles of the humeral head that occurs in a tear of the rotator cuff or biceps tendon as the principal cause of secondary impingement. Where a defective rotator cuff is no longer able to counterbalance the superior pull of the deltoid, elevating the shoulder will cause the humeral head to shift upwards and produce impingement. The same also applies to shoulder instability, where, especially in multidirectional displacement, the humeral head is pulled against the roof of the joint capsule, producing impingement. Functional constriction can also result where muscular paralysis and weakness prevent involvement of the scapula in the overall elevation of the arm, or where separation of the acromioclavicular joint has eliminated its supporting structures. Finally, one should also remember the pathogenetic significance of a shrunken posterior capsule. If the humeral head cannot glide far enough posteriorly in flexion, it will be increasingly pressed against the anterior margin of the acromion, resulting in impingement.

The chronic stage of impingement syndrome can involve clinically conspicuous deltoid atrophy as well as supraspinatus and infraspinatus atrophy. The tendon insertions on the greater and lesser tubercles of the humerus are often tender to palpation, and mobility in the glenohumeral joint is often limited toward the end of its range of motion. Active elevation is more painful than passive elevation.

Where the patient is able to abduct his or her arm against resistance in spite of pain, this suggests degenerative tendon changes rather than a tear. The Neer impingement injection test allows one to clinically distinguish between weakness in abduction due to a rupture and that due to pain. In the presence of a tendon rupture, the weakness in abducting the arm may be expected to remain even after infiltration of the subacromial space with anesthetic has reduced or eliminated pain.

A patient with "pseudo-paralysis" is unable to lift the affected arm. This global sign suggests a rotator cuff disorder. Further examinations are then required to identify the damaged tendon. Provocative tests can be very helpful in this regard. External and internal rotation against resistance is evaluated with the shoulder in various positions. Weakness is more probably due to a functional deficit (such as a rupture), whereas pain is more probably attributable to inflammation of the tendon insertions or the adjacent bursae.

## Zero-Degree Abduction Test

**Procedure:**   The patient is standing with his or her arms hanging relaxed. The examiner grasps the distal third of each forearm. The patient attempts to abduct the arms against the examiner's resistance.

**Assessment:**   Abduction of the arm is initiated by the supraspinatus and deltoid. Pain and, especially, weakness in abducting and holding the arm strongly suggest a rotator cuff tear.

Eccentricity of the humeral head in the form of superior displacement of the humeral head in a rotator cuff tear causes relative insufficiency of the outer muscles of the shoulder. Small tears that can be functionally compensated for will cause minor loss of function with the same amount of pain. Larger tears are invariably characterized by weakness and loss of function.

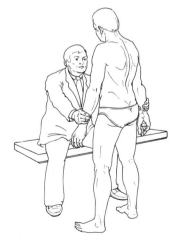

Fig. **2.8**   Zero-Degree abduction test

## Jobe Supraspinatus Test

**Procedure:**    This test may be performed with the patient standing or seated.

With the elbow extended, the patient's arm is held at 90° of abduction, 30° of horizontal flexion, and in internal-neutral and external rotation. The examiner exerts pressure on the upper arm during the abduction and horizontal flexion motion. The supraspinatus can be tested largely in isolation after electromyography. It is important to apply pressure gently at first and increase the pressure if the patient does not have pain.

**Assessment:**    When this test elicits severe pain and the patient is unable to hold his or her arm abducted 90° against gravity, this is called a positive drop arm sign.

The superior portions of the rotator cuff (supraspinatus) are particularly assessed in internal rotation (with the thumb down as when emptying a can), and the anterior portions in external rotation.

The test may be repeated at only 45° abduction to differentiate findings. Where the impingement component predominates, there will be less pain and more strength where the tendon is still intact. The test can yield false-positive results where pathology of the long head of the biceps tendon is present.

Where the test elicits pain and the patient is unable to abduct the arm 90° and hold it against gravity, this indicates a tear of the supraspinatus tendon, or muscle, or neuropathy of the suprascapular nerve.

Strength in the supraspinatus muscle may not be diminished until over two-thirds of the tendon is torn.

Injection studies into the suprascapular and axillary nerves substantiate that both the supraspinatus and deltoid muscle function in elevation of the arm.

Therefore, the supraspinatus tendon can be completely torn and the shoulder can have full range of motion. The only deficit will be weakness using the arm for lifting above shoulder level and with the arm away from the body.

EMG tests show no difference in the EMG activity with the arm in full internal rotation (classic Jobe *empty can* position) with the thumb parallel to the floor and with the arm in maximum external rotation (*full can* position).

The strength of the supraspinatus muscle can also be tested with the elbows flexed rather than extended to decrease the stress. It is less painful for patients.

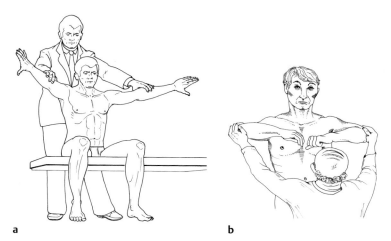

Fig. 2.**9a, b**
**a** Jobe supraspinatus test,
**b** Jobe supraspinatus test with elbow flexed. Abduction of the arm to 90°, the elbow is flexed

### Subscapularis Test

**Procedure:**   This test has the opposite effect with respect to the infraspinatus. With the patient's elbow alongside but not quite touching the trunk, the examiner comparatively assesses passive external rotation in both arms and active internal rotation of the shoulder against resistance.

**Assessment:**   Increased painless passive external rotation in comparison with the contralateral side and weakness of the active internal rotation suggests an isolated tear of the subscapularis.

A tear of the subscapularis manifests itself as pain and weakness in internal rotation. Where pain is slight, this reduced strength suggests a tear. Where pain is more severe, it is not usually possible to distinguish between a tear and tendinopathy.

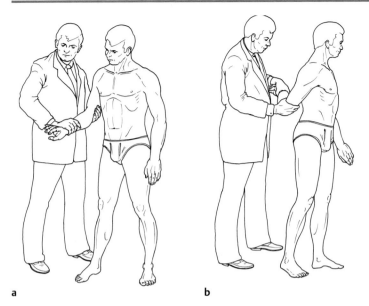

Fig. **2.10a, b**   Subscapularis test:
**a** passive external rotation,
**b** active internal rotation behind the back

## Gerber Lift-Off Test

**Procedure:**   The patient places the dorsum of the hand on his or her back with the arm in internal rotation. The patient then lifts the hand away from the back. If the patient is able to take the hand away from the back, the examiner should apply a load, pushing the hand toward the back to test the strength of the subscapularis and to test how the scapula acts under dynamic loading.

**Assessment:**   Where a tendon rupture or insufficiency of the subscapularis is present, the patient will be unable to lift the hand off the back against the examiner's resistance. Where pain renders maximum internal rotation impossible, the belly press test may be performed.

With a torn subscapularis tendon, passive (and active) lateral rotation will increase. If the patient's hand is passively medially rotated as far as possible and the patient is asked to hold the position, the examiner will note that the hand moves toward the back (subscapularis or

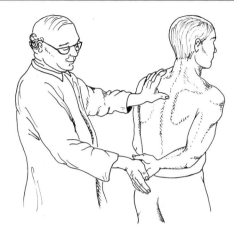

Fig. 2.**11**   Lift-off test

medial rotation *spring back* or leg test) as the subscapularis cannot hold the position due to weakness or pain. This test is also called the modified lift-off-test.

A short lag between maximum passive medial rotation and active medial rotation suggests a partial tear of the subscapularis. This modified test is reported to be more accurate in diagnosing rotator cuff tear. The test may also be used to test the rhomboids. Medial border winging of the scapula during the test may indicate that the rhomboids are affected.

Because many patients with biceps subluxations have partial or full-thickness tears of the subscapularis, a positive test may indicate not only subscapularis, but also biceps tendon pathology. Where pain renders maximum internal rotation impossible, the Napoleon sign may be performed.

## Belly Press–Abdominal Compression Test

**Procedure:**  The patient is standing. The patient's forearm lies along the abdomen with the elbow flexed. The patient attempts to continue forcefully pressing arm against abdomen.

**Assessment:**  A tear in the supraspinatus tendon results in loss of the internal rotation component. The elbow deviates laterally and posteriorly under the influence of the latissimus dorsi and teres major. Flexion also occurs in the wrist.

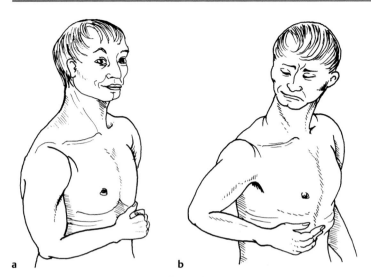

Fig. 2.**12a, b**    Belly press test–abdominal compression test:
**a**  the forearm lies along the abdomen with the elbow flexed,
**b**  the arm deviates laterally and posteriorly while the wrist is flexed

## Napoleon Sign

The active and passive lift-off test is only allowed where free active and passive internal rotation is possible in the injured shoulder.

**Procedure:** The patient is instructed to press the palm of his or her hand against the abdomen.

**Assessment:** Normally these motions produce anterior motion in the elbow due to the tension in the subscapularis musculature. In patients with a rupture in the subscapularis tendon, the position of the arm remains unchanged. Some patients also exhibit increased passive external rotation.

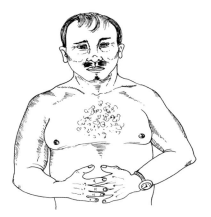

Fig. 2.**13** Napoleon sign: both hands are pressed against the abdomen

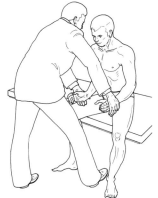

Fig. 2.**14** Infraspinatus test

### Infraspinatus Test

**Procedure:** This test may be performed with the patient seated or standing.

Comparative testing of both sides is best. The patient's arms should hang relaxed with the elbows flexed 90° but not quite touching the trunk. The examiner places his or her palms on the dorsum of each of the patient's hands and then asks the patient to externally rotate both forearms against the resistance of the examiner's hands.

**Assessment:** Pain or weakness in external rotation indicates a disorder of the infraspinatus (external rotator). As infraspinatus tears are usually painless, weakness in rotation strongly suggests a tear in this muscle. This test can also be performed with the arm abducted 90° and flexed 30° to eliminate involvement of the deltoid in this motion. The most common etiology for the atrophy of the infraspinatus is tendon tears or damage to the infraspinatus branch of the suprascapular nerve by compressive lesions (synovial cyst) or by traction injuries (overhead athletes, volleyball players).

The infraspinatus fills the infraspinatus fossa of the scapula. The best way to demonstrate infraspinatus atrophy is to ask the patient to undress. Compression toward the contralateral side is helpful in determining if changes are unilateral or bilateral.

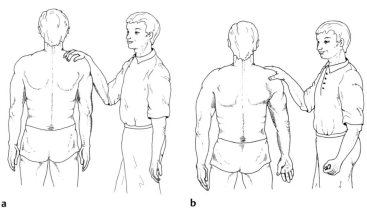

**a**                                        **b**

Fig. 2.**15a, b**   Teres test:
**a** normal position,
**b** contracture in the right arm

## Teres Test

**Procedure:**   The patient is standing and relaxed. The examiner assesses the position of the patient's hands from behind.

**Assessment:**   The teres major is an internal rotator. Where a contracture is present, the palm of the affected hand will face backward compared with the contralateral hand. With the patient standing in a relaxed position, such a finding suggests a contracture of the teres major.

Weakness of the rotator cuff or a brachial plexus lesion can also produce an asymmetrical hand position.

## Abduction External Rotation Test

**Procedure:**   The arm is abducted 90° and flexed 30°. This neutralizes the effect of the deltoid in external rotation. The patient attempts to continue to externally rotate the arm against the resistance of the examiner's hand.

**Assessment:**   The lack of active external rotation in the abducted arm suggests a clinically significant rupture of the infraspinatus tendon.

Performing the test at over 45° of external rotation primarily tests the teres minor.

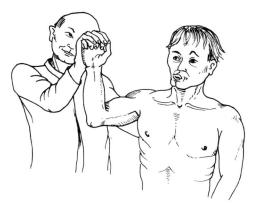

Fig. 2.**16** Abduction external rotation test

## Nonspecific Supraspinatus Test

**Procedure:** The patient is seated with the arm abducted 90° with the examiner's hand resting on the patient's forearm. The examiner then asks the patient to further abduct the arm against the examiner's resistance.

**Assessment:** Weakness in further abduction and/or pain indicate pathology of the supraspinatus tendon.

**Note:** Painful arc syndrome is sometimes confused with arthritis of the acromioclavicular joint, which also causes pain during a certain phase of the abduction arc.

## Drop Arm Test

**Procedure:** The patient is seated and the extended arm passively abducted 90°. The patient is instructed to hold the arm in this position without support and then slowly lower it.

**Assessment:** Weakness in maintaining the position of the arm, with or without pain, or sudden dropping of the arm suggests a rotator cuff lesion. Most often this is due to a defect in the supraspinatus. In pseudoparalysis, the patient will be unable to lift the affected arm. This global sign suggests a rotator cuff disorder.

A painless drop arm sign can also be seen in neurologic diseases. Therefore patients with a positive drop arm sign should be examined carefully for such findings.

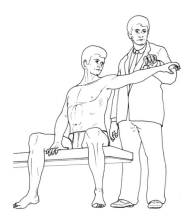

Fig. 2.**17**   Drop arm test

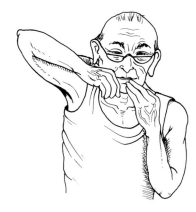

Fig. 2.**18**   Hornblower sign

### Walch Hornblower Sign

**Procedure:**   The patient is requested to touch his or her mouth with the affected hand.

**Assessment:**   Where there is complete insufficiency of both external rotators (infraspinatus and teres minor), the arm will deviate into internal rotation and the patient will have to lift the elbow higher than the hand. To reach their mouth, they must first elevate the arm to about 90°. This allows the weak arm to fall into internal rotation, so that the arm assumes a position resembling a person blowing a horn. The sensitivity and specificity of this sign is very high.

### Apley's Scratch Test

**Procedure:**   The seated patient is asked to touch the contralateral superior medial corner of the scapula with the index finger.

**Assessment:**   Pain elicited in the rotator cuff and failure to reach the scapula because of restricted mobility in external rotation and abduction indicate rotator cuff pathology (most probably involving the supraspinatus). A differential diagnosis should consider osteoarthritis in the glenohumeral and acromioclavicular joints as well as capsular fibrosis.

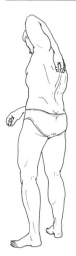

Fig. 2.**19**   Apley's scratch test

## Painful Arc

**Procedure:**   The arm is passively and actively abducted from the rest position alongside the trunk.

**Assessment:**   Pain occurring in abduction between 70° and 120° (Fig. 2.**20a**) is a sign of a lesion of the supraspinatus tendon, which becomes impinged between the greater tubercle of the humerus and the acromion in this phase of the motion (subacromial impingement). (Contrast this with the painful arc in acromioclavicular joint disorders, where the pain only occurs only at 140°–180° of abduction, Fig. 2.**20c**; see also Fig. 2.**24**). Patients are usually free of pain above 120°.

In the evaluation of the active and passive ranges of motion, the patient can often avoid the painful arc by externally rotating the arm while abducting it. This increases the clearance between the acromion and the diseased tendinous portion of the rotator cuff, avoiding impingement in the range between 70° and 120°.

In addition to complete or incomplete rotator cuff tears, swelling and inflammation as a result of bursitis and abnormality of the margin of the acromion occasionally lead to impingement with a painful arc, as does osteoarthritis in the acromioclavicular joint.

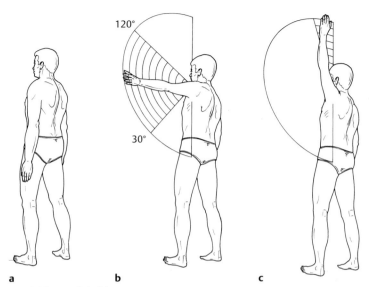

Fig. 2.**20a–c**   Painful arc:
**a** starting position,
**b** painful motion between 30° and 120°,
**c** pain at the end of the range of motion, a sign of acromioclavicular joint pathology

## Neer Impingement Sign

**Procedure:**   The examiner immobilizes the scapula with one hand while the other hand jerks the patient's arm forward, upward, and sideways (medially) into the scapular plane.

**Assessment:**   If an impingement syndrome is present, subacromial constriction or impingement of the diseased area against the anterior inferior margin of the acromion will produce severe pain with motion. The impingement sign is nonspecific and can produce pain from a variety of conditions (bursitis, stiffness, anterior instability, arthritis, calcific tendonitis, bone lesions, rotator cuff tears). If the test is positive when done with the arm laterally rotated, the examiner should check the acromioclavicular joint (acromioclavicular differentiation test).

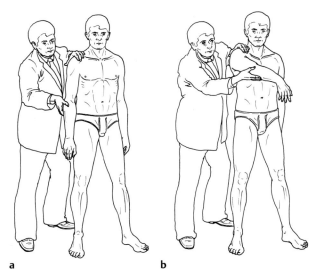

**a**                          **b**

Fig. 2.**21a, b**  Neer impingement sign:
**a** starting position,
**b** forcible forward flexion and adduction of the extended arm

## Hawkins and Kennedy Impingement Test

**Procedure:**  The examiner immobilizes the scapula with one hand while the other hand adducts the patient's 90°-forward-flexed and internally rotated arm (moving it toward the contralateral side of the body).

**Assessment:**  Pain indicates a positive test for supraspinatus peritendinitis, tendinitis, or secondary impingement.

In a positive impingement syndrome, impingement of the greater tubercle or compression of the supraspinatus tendon occurs, causing severe pain on motion. Coracoid impingement is revealed by the adduction motion, in which the supraspinatus tendon also impinges against the coracoid process.

In the Jobe impingement test, the forward flexed and slightly adducted arm is forcibly internally rotated. This will provoke typical impingement pain.

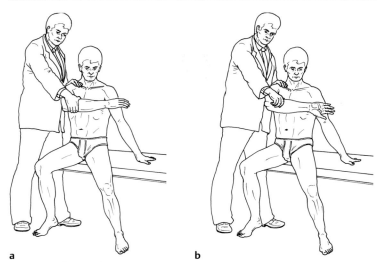

**a**                                   **b**

Fig. 2.**22a, b**   Hawkins impingement sign:
**a** starting position
**b** forcible internal rotation (Jobe)

## Neer Impingement Injection Test

**Procedure:**   The region beneath the anterior acromion or the subacromial space is infiltrated with an anesthetic. To open the subacromial space, the patient is asked to sit on the side of the table with the arm hanging down unsupported. The weight of the arm will open the subacromial space only if the patient is relaxed. The injection should be done with sterile technique.

**Caution:**   After the injection it is necessary to observe the patient for vasovagal symptoms. Patients are warned about potential side effects including pain and loss of motion briefly after the injection and that the shoulder may be sore for a few days (especially after combined anesthetic and corticosteroid injection).

**Assessment:**   This test allows the examiner to determine whether subacromial impingement is the cause of the painful arc. A painful arc that disappears or improves after the injection is caused by changes in the subacromial space, such as bursitis or an activated rotator cuff defect.

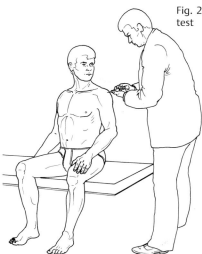

Fig. 2.**23** Neer impingement injection test

# Acromioclavicular Joint

The acromial end of the clavicle articulates with the acromion. The acromioclavicular ligament reinforces the capsule of this joint. Functionally, the articulation is a ball-and-socket joint whose range of motion is less than that of the sternoclavicular joint. Another strong ligament joins the scapula and clavicle, the coracoclavicular ligament. It arises from the coracoid process and inserts into the inferior aspect of the clavicle. One of the most helpful signs of the presence of acromioclavicular joint problems is to compare the two shoulders for asymmetry of the acromioclavicular joints (e. g., asymptomatic arthritis, trauma, tumors, infections, synovial cysts).

Osteoarthritis of the acromioclavicular joint can cause pain and further constrict the subacromial space. In addition to pain with motion and tenderness to palpation over the shoulder, palpation will often reveal thickening of the bony joint margins.

The vast majority of degenerative acromioclavicular joints are not symptomatic and do not warrant treatment.

Acromioclavicular joint disease can also mimic cervical spine disease (which frequently radiates down the trapezius into the superior shoulder), a superior labrum anterior and posterior (SLAP) lesion, and a rotator cuff disease.

Acromioclavicular capsular ligament injures are common. Rockwood classified acromioclavicular joint injuries in six grades.

**Grade 1:** Acromioclavicular joint sprain

**Grade 2:** Partial rupture of the acromioclavicular and coracoclavicular ligaments and subluxation in the acromioclavicular joint

**Grade 3:** Complete rupture of the acromioclavicular and coracoclavicular ligaments, dislocation of the acromioclavicular joint

**Grade 4:** Dislocation of the acromioclavicular joint, the clavicle is posteriorly displaced into the trapezius

**Grade 5:** Dislocation of the acromioclavicular joint, the clavicle is superiorly displaced by at least twice the width of the clavicle

**Grade 6:** Dislocation of the acromioclavicular joint, the clavicle is inferiorly displaced beneath the coracoid process

## Painful Arc

**Procedure:**   The patient's arm is passively and actively abducted from the rest position alongside the trunk.

**Assessment:**   Pain in the acromioclavicular joint occurs between 140° and 180° of abduction. Increasing abduction leads to increasing com-

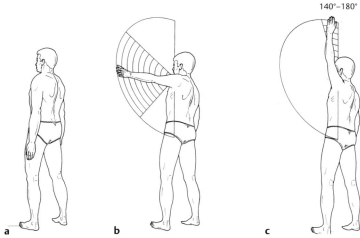

Fig. 2.**24a–c**   Painful arc:
**a** starting position,
**b** pain between 30° and 120°(sign of a supraspinatus syndrome),
**c** pain between 140° and 180° (sign of osteoarthritis in the acromioclavicular joint)

pression and contortion in the joint. (In an impingement syndrome or a rotator cuff tear, by comparison, pain symptoms will occur between 70° and 120°; see Fig. 2.**20**).

## Crossed Body Adduction Stress Test

**Procedure:**   The 90°-abducted arm on the affected side is forcibly adducted across the chest toward the normal side.

**Assessment:**   Pain in the acromioclavicular joint suggests joint pathology or anterior impingement. (Absence of pain after injection of an anesthetic is a sign of joint disease.)

## Forced Adduction Test on Hanging Arm

**Procedure:**   The examiner grasps the upper arm of the affected side with one hand while the other hand rests on the contralateral shoulder and immobilizes the shoulder girdle. Then the examiner forcibly adducts the hanging affected arm behind the patient's back against the patient's resistance.

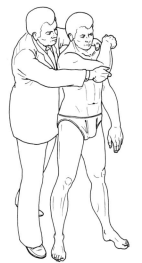

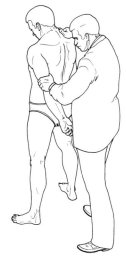

Fig. 2.**25**   Crossed body adduction stress test

Fig. 2.**26**   Forced adduction test on hanging arm

**Assessment:** Pain across the anterior aspect of the shoulder suggests acromioclavicular joint disease or subacromial impingement. (Symptoms that disappear or improve following injection of an anesthetic indicate that the acromioclavicular joint is causing the pain.)

## Clavicle Mobility Test

**Procedure:** The examiner grasps the lateral end of the clavicle between two fingers and moves it in every direction.

**Assessment:** Increased mobility of the lateral clavicle with or without pain is a sign of instability in the acromioclavicular joint. In isolated osteoarthritis there will be circumscribed tenderness to palpation and pain with motion. Acromioclavicular joint separation with rupture of the coracoclavicular ligaments will be accompanied by a positive "piano key" sign: the subluxated lateral end of the clavicle displaces proximally with the pull of the cervical musculature and can be pressed inferiorly against elastic resistance.

## Dugas Test

**Procedure:** The patient is seated or standing and touches the contralateral shoulder with the hand of the 90°-flexed arm of the affected side.

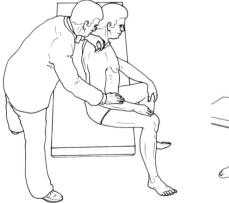

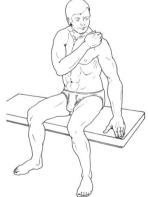

Fig. 2.**27**   Clavicle mobility test          Fig. 2.**28**   Dugas test

**Assessment:** Acromioclavicular joint pain suggests joint disease (osteoarthritis, instability, disk injury, or infection). A differential diagnosis must exclude anterior subacromial impingement, due to the topographic proximity of that region.

### Acromioclavicular Injection Test

**Procedure:** Inject the acromioclavicular joint with an anesthetic such as lidocaine (with a corticosteroid where indicated). A sterile preparation of the area is applied prior to the injection and the injection is done with sterile technique. Large osteophytes, arthritic joints, and an impinged meniscus render injection difficult.

**Assessment:** Where injection relieves local pain, isolated acromioclavicular pathology is present. To confirm the diagnosis it is recommended to attempt to reproduce the pain with whatever examination produced the most pain prior to injection, such as a cross arm adduction test or painful arc.

## ■ Long Head of the Biceps Tendon

A rupture of the long head of the biceps tendon will appear as a distally displaced protrusion of the muscle belly of the biceps. The close anatomic proximity of the intraarticular portion of the tendon to the coracoacromial arch predisposes it to involvement in degenerative processes in the subacromial space. A rotator cuff tear is often accompanied by a rupture of the long head of the biceps tendon.

Isolated inflammation of the long head of the biceps tendon (bicipital tenosynovitis) is accordingly rare. In younger patients, this may occur as a tennis or throwing injury. Subluxations of the long head of the biceps tendon in the bicipital groove are usually difficult to detect. However, a series of specific tests can be used to diagnose biceps tendon injuries; the typical sign of these injuries is not the distally displaced muscle belly but incomplete contraction and/or "snapping" of the tendon.

### Nonspecific Biceps Tendon Test

**Procedure:** The patient holds the arm abducted in neutral rotation with the elbow flexed 90°. The examiner immobilizes the patient's elbow with one hand and places the heel of the other hand on the patient's distal forearm. The patient is then asked to externally rotate his or her arm against the resistance of the examiner's hand.

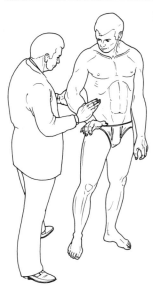

Fig. 2.**29**   Nonspecific biceps tendon test

**Assessment:**   Pain in the bicipital groove or at the insertion of the biceps suggests a tendon disorder.

Pain in the anterolateral aspect of the shoulder is often a sign of a disorder of the rotator cuff, especially the infraspinatus tendon.

### Abbott–Saunders Test

Demonstrates subluxation of the long head of the biceps tendon in the bicipital groove.

**Procedure:**   The patient's arm is externally rotated and abducted about 120° with progressive internal rotation. The examiner slowly lowers the arm from this position. The examiner guides this motion of the patient's arm with one hand while resting the other on the patient's shoulder and palpating the bicipital groove with the index and middle fingers.

**Assessment:**   Pain in the region of the bicipital groove or a palpable or audible snap suggest a disorder of the biceps tendon (subluxation sign). An inflamed bursa (subcoracoid or subscapular bursa) can also occasionally cause snapping.

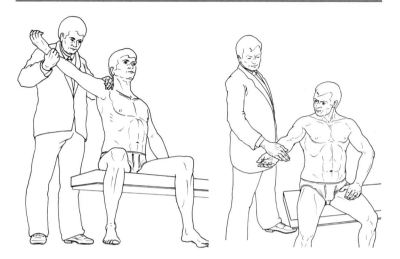

Fig. 2.**30**  Abbott–Saunders test    Fig. 2.**31**  Speed test

## Palm-Up Test (Speed Biceps or Straight Arm Test)

**Procedure:**  The patient's arm is extended in supination at 90° of abduction and 30° of horizontal flexion. The patient attempts to either maintain this position or continue to abduct and pronate the arm against the downward pressure of the examiner's hand.

**Assessment:**  A positive test elicits increased tenderness in the bicipital groove especially with the arm supinated and is indicative of bicipital paratenonitis or tendinosis.

## Snap Test

Tests for subluxation of the long head of the biceps tendon.

**Procedure:**  The examiner palpates the bicipital groove with the index and middle finger of one hand. With the other hand, the examiner grasps the wrist of the patient's arm (abducted 80°–90° and flexed 90° at the elbow) and passively rotates it at the shoulder, first in one direction and then the other.

**Assessment:**  Subluxation of the long head of the biceps tendon out of the bicipital groove will be detectable as a palpable snap.

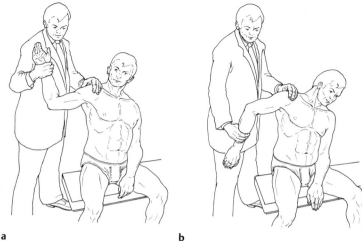

**a**                                    **b**

Fig. 2.**32a, b**  Snap test:
**a** external rotation,
**b** internal rotation

### Yergason Test

Functional test of the long head of the biceps tendon.

**Procedure:**  The patient's arm is alongside the trunk and flexed 90° at the elbow. One of the examiner's hands rests on the patient's shoulder and palpates the bicipital groove with the index finger while the other hand grasps the patient's forearm. The patient is asked to supinate the forearm against the examiner's resistance. This places isolated tension on the long head of the biceps tendon.

**Assessment:**  Pain in the bicipital groove is a sign of a lesion of the biceps tendon, its tendon sheath, or its ligamentous connection via the transverse ligament. The typical provoked pain can be increased by pressing on the tendon in the bicipital groove.

### Hueter Sign

**Procedure:**  The patient is seated with the arm extended at the elbow and the forearm in supination. The examiner grasps the posterior aspect of the patient's forearm. The patient is then asked to flex the elbow against the resistance of the examiner's hand.

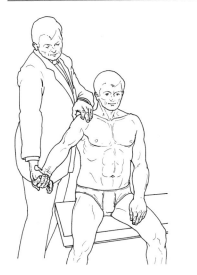

Fig. 2.**33** Yergason test

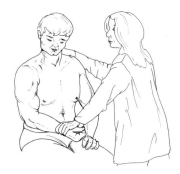

Fig. 2.**34** Hueter sign

**Assessment:** In a rupture of the long head of the biceps tendon, the distally displaced muscle belly can be observed as a "ball" directly proximal to the elbow.

### Transverse Humeral Ligament Test

**Procedure:** The patient is seated with the arm abducted 90°, internally rotated, and extended at the elbow. From this position, the examiner externally rotates the arm while palpating the bicipital groove to verify whether the tendon snaps.

**Assessment:** In the presence of ligamentous insufficiency, this motion will cause the biceps tendon to spontaneously displace out of the bicipital groove. Pain reported without displacement suggests biceps tendinitis.

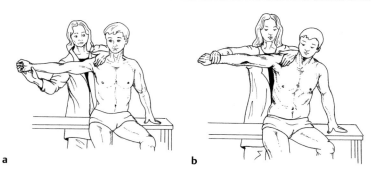

Fig. 2.**35a, b**    Transverse humeral ligament test:
**a** starting position,
**b** palpating the biceps tendon in internal rotation

## Thompson and Kopell Horizontal Flexion Test (Cross-Body Action)

**Procedure:**    The patient is standing and moves the 90°-abducted arm across the body into maximum horizontal flexion.

**Assessment:**    Dull, deep-seated pain above the superior margin of the scapula in the supraspinatus fossa and on the posterolateral scapula radiating into the upper arm can be caused by compression of the suprascapular nerve beneath the transverse scapular ligament as a result of distal displacement of the scapula.

**Note:**    A differential diagnosis must consider pain due to acromioclavicular joint pathology. Such pain can also be elicited by this test maneuver.

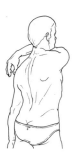

Fig. 2.**36**    Thompson and Kopell horizontal flexion test

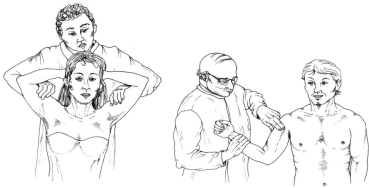

Fig. 2.**37**   Ludington test: the patient places both hands behind the head, testing the biceps tendon

Fig. 2.**38**   Lippmann test: the arm is flexed to 90°; the examiner palpates the biceps tendon

## Ludington Test

**Procedure:**   The patient is standing and is asked to place both hands behind the head locking the fingers. This allows the arms to be supported by the hands on the head and allows the biceps to relax. The patient then is asked to relax and contract the biceps tendon. The examiner stands behind the patient and palpates the proximal biceps tendon to see if tension is found in the tendon with muscle contraction.

**Assessment:**   If there is no tension in the tendon, then the proximal biceps tendon may be torn.

## Lippman Test

**Procedure:**   The patient is sitting or standing, and the examiner is holding the arm of the patient flexed to 90 degrees. The examiner palpates the biceps tendon in the bicipital groove 6 to 8 cm below the glenohumeral joint und attempts to move it back and forth.

**Assessment:**   If the patient feels a sharp pain in the biceps tendon when it is being flipped back and forth, then tendon pathology is present.

## SLAP Lesions

The intraarticular insertion of the long head of the biceps tendon forms an integral unit with the adjacent superior glenoid labrum. A fall on the extended, slightly flexed, and abducted arm; trauma in external rotation and abduction; and microtrauma from repeated throwing motions can all lead to superior labral-anterior posterior (SLAP) lesions. Associated injuries are common and may include tears of the rotator cuff and Bankart lesions.

Snyder classifies SLAP lesions as follows:

**Type I:**   (11%) Labral degeneration not affecting the margin of the labrum or biceps anchor.

**Type II:**   (41%) Avulsion of the biceps tendon from the supraglenoid tubercle. Biceps and labrum are avulsed together. Anterior, posterior, or combined lesion.

**Type III:**   (33%) Bucket-handle tears of the superior labrum with intact biceps anchor.

**Type IV:**   (15%) Bucket handle tear of the superior labrum involving the biceps anchor.

## O'Brien Active Compression Test

Assessment of a superior labral-anterior posterior (SLAP) lesion. Separation of the glenoid labrum from the anterior superior and posterior superior margins of the glenoid accompanied by avulsion of the insertion of the long head of the biceps tendon.

**Procedure:**   The patient stands with the elbow extended and moves his or her arm into 90° flexion, 10° adduction, and maximum internal rotation (thumbs pointing downward). The examiner attempts to press

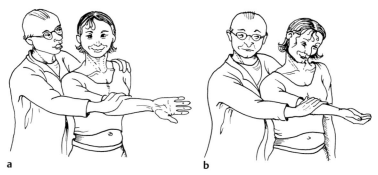

a                              b

Fig. 2.**39a, b**   O'Brien active compression test

the arm downward against the patient's resistance (the test is then repeated in maximum external rotation).

**Assessment:**   The test is positive where the first phase elicits pain that then lessens or disappears in supination (maximum external rotation). It is crucial to inquire about the location of the pain as the O'Brien test can also yield positive results in the presence of acromioclavicular joint disorders. Pain reported within the shoulder suggests a SLAP lesion, whereas pain over the acromioclavicular joint may also be due to osteoarthritis of the acromioclavicular joint.

In addition to the O'Brien test, the internal rotation resistance strength test (IRRS test) is suitable for clinical evaluation of the biceps tendon insertion. In this test, the patient moves his or her arm with the elbow flexed into 90° abduction and 80° external rotation. The patient is then asked to rotate the arm externally and then internally against the examiner's resistance. The test is positive where the strength of internal rotation is significantly less than that of external rotation.

The active compression test is a test for both acromioclavicular joint problems and SLAP lesions. When the test is performed, the patient is asked whether the pain provoked when his palm is down (the first half of the test) is located on top of the shoulder near the acromioclavicular joint or if it is located deep in the joint. If the pain is superficial, this indicates an acromioclavicular joint problem; if it is deep in the joint, it is suspicious for a SLAP lesion. The test is repeated with the palm up, and the pain should be diminished regardless of the etiology.

### Biceps Load Test 1

Diagnosis of superior labrum tears in patients who had anterior shoulder instability associated with Bankart lesions.

**Procedure:**   The patient is placed supine and the extremity abducted to 90 degrees. The elbow is flexed 90° and the arm is placed in a neutral rotation. The forearm is supinated and then an anterior apprehension maneuver is performed.

When the patient becomes apprehensive, external rotation is stopped. The patient is then asked to actively flex the forearm at the elbow by bringing the hand toward his face. Upon resistance by the examiner, the patient is asked if the feeling of instability is improved, unchanged, or worsened.

**Assessment:**   If the pain is unimproved or worsens, then there is suspicion of a SLAP lesion. The examiner should note that the forearm should be supinated during the test. Also, the examiner should be at the same level as the patient, e. g., sitting on a chair.

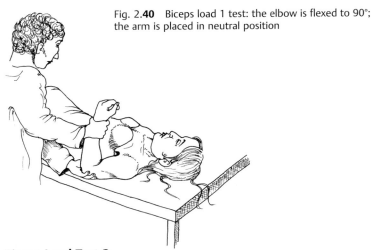

Fig. 2.**40**    Biceps load 1 test: the elbow is flexed to 90°; the arm is placed in neutral position

## Biceps Load Test 2

Test for isolated SLAP lesions independent of shoulder instability

**Procedure:**  The rationale for the test is that resisted flexion of the arm with the forearm in a supinated position places stress on the proximal biceps anchor.

The patient is supine, but the arm is abducted to 120° of elevation. The arm is then externally rotated to its maximal extent, and the elbow is flexed 90° and the forearm supinated. The patient is asked to flex the elbow toward the head while the examiner resists that motion.

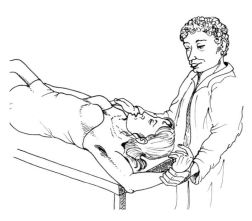

Fig. 2.**41**    Biceps load 2 test: the arm is abducted to 120° and rotated to its maximal extent. The elbow is flexed to 90°

**Assessment:** A positive test is the presence of pain with the test or increased pain over baseline with the test. A negative test is the absence of pain or a lack of increase in the baseline pain.

# ■ Shoulder Instability

The joint capsule of the shoulder may be too loose, leading to instability. Often this is attributable to congenital generalized laxity of the ligaments (hyperlaxity) with increased bilateral multidirectional instability. Chronic shoulder pain may be attributable to an unstable shoulder. The clinical picture of subluxation in particular is often difficult to diagnose, and patients themselves can usually give only a vague description of their symptoms.

According to Neer, instability patients invariably have a history of a period of intensive shoulder use (such as competitive sports), an episode of repeated minor trauma (overhead use), or generalized ligament laxity. Both young athletes and inactive persons are affected, men and women alike.

The transition between subluxation and dislocation is continuous. There is no clearly defined point before which a lesion is still a subluxation and beyond which it is already a dislocation. Patients with voluntary instability are a separate issue. In such cases, consultation with a psychologist may be helpful in addition to repeated clinical examination.

The differential diagnosis must specifically consider an impingement syndrome, a rotator cuff tear, osteoarthritis in the acromioclavicular joint, and also a cervical spine syndrome. In cases of doubt, injection of a local anesthetic at the point of maximum pain may be required.

However, this treatment cannot permanently eliminate instability symptoms. Signs of generalized ligament laxity may include increased mobility in other joints and, especially, increased hyperextension in the elbow or retroflexion in the metacarpophalangeal joint of the thumb with the forearm extended. The use of a variety of relatively specific tests will make it easier for the examiner to arrive at a diagnosis.

Assessment of the range of motion is crucial in patients with suspected shoulder instability. Rotation should be examined in both adduction and 90°-abduction. Restricted external rotation in both adduction and abduction will often be the first sign of instability in patients with anterior instability. Flexion and abduction in the scapular plane are not normally restricted.

## Compression Test

**Procedure and assessment:**   Passive elevation of the arm to the end of its range of motion with continued application of posterior pressure produces pain as a result of compression of the biceps tendon between the acromion and humeral head.

Evaluation of the range of motion is crucial in patients with suspected shoulder instability. Rotation should be examined both in adduction and 90°-abduction. Restricted external rotation in both adduction and abduction will often be the first sign of instability in patients with anterior instability. Flexion and abduction in the scapular plane are not normally restricted.

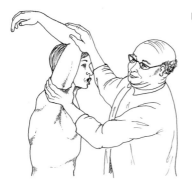

Fig. 2.**42**    Compression test

## Anterior Apprehension Test

*Tests of shoulder stability.*

**Procedure:**   The examination begins with the patient seated. The examiner palpates the humeral head through the surrounding soft tissue with one hand and guides the patient's arm with the other hand. The examiner passively abducts the patient's shoulder with the elbow flexed and then brings the shoulder into maximum external rotation, keeping the arm in this position. The test is performed at 60°, 90°, and 120° of abduction to evaluate the superior, medial, and inferior glenohumeral ligaments. With the guiding hand, the examiner presses the humeral head in an anterior and inferior direction.

The examiner then applies a posterior translational stress to the head of the humerus or the arm, and the patient will commonly lose the

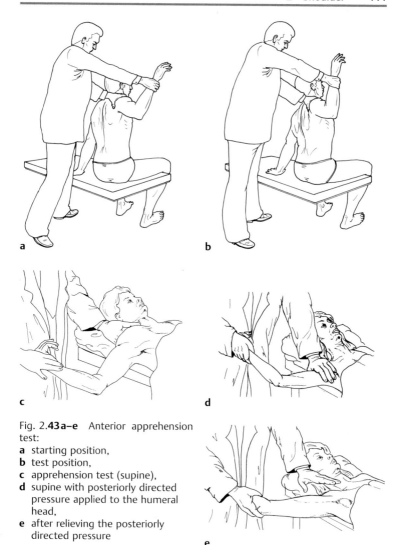

Fig. 2.**43a–e** Anterior apprehension test:
**a** starting position,
**b** test position,
**c** apprehension test (supine),
**d** supine with posteriorly directed pressure applied to the humeral head,
**e** after relieving the posteriorly directed pressure

apprehension. Any pain that is present commonly decreases and further lateral rotation is possible before the apprehension and/or pain returns.

The test is considered positive if pain decreases during the maneuver even if there was no apprehension (Fowler sign or Jobe relocation test).

**Note:** The test must be performed slowly. If the test is done too quickly, there is a chance that the humeral head will dislocate.

**Assessment:** Shoulder pain with reflexive muscle tensing is a sign of an anterior instability syndrome. This muscle tension is an attempt by the patient to prevent imminent subluxation or dislocation of the humeral head. Even without pain and with tension only in the anterior shoulder musculature (pectoralis), there may be signs of instability.

Placing the patient supine improves the specificity of the apprehension test. By placing the left hand under the glenohumeral joint to act as a fulcrum the apprehension test becomes a fulcrum test.

In a further stage of the apprehension test, releasing the posteriorly directed pressure causes a sudden increase in pain with the apprehension phenomenon (release test).

In a modification by Jobe, the apprehension phenomenon can also be specified in four grades of severity (impingement and instability often occur together).

**Grade 1:**   Pure impingement with no instability

**Grade 2:**   Secondary instability and instability caused by chronic capsular and labral microtrauma

**Grade 3:**   Secondary impingement and instability caused by generalized hypermobility or laxity

**Grade 4:**   Primary instability with no impingement

Applying increasing posterior pressure to the humeral head increases the pain and dislocation sensation in the same manner as increasing external rotation and abduction.

**Note:** Hawkins describes a three-grade system for anterior translation (Fig. 2.**44**).

**Note:** When the patient complains of sudden stabbing pain with simultaneous or subsequent paralyzing weakness in the affected extremity, this is referred to as the "dead arm sign." It is attributable to the transient compression the subluxated humeral head exerts on the plexus.

It is important to know that at 45° of abduction, the test primarily evaluates the medial glenohumeral ligament and the subscapularis tendon. At or above 90° of abduction, the stabilizing effect of the subscapularis is neutralized and the test primarily evaluates the inferior glenohumeral ligament.

The Hawkins classification of instability is based upon what is felt by the examiner.

**Grade 0:**   normal laxity (amount of translation)
**Grade 1:**   humeral head moves slightly up to the glenoid rim
**Grade 2:**   humeral head rides over the rim, but spontaneously reduces
**Grade 3:**   humeral head rides up and over the glenoid rim, but remains dislocated

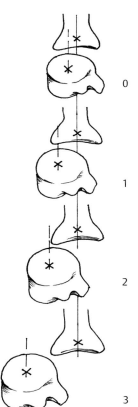

Fig. 2.**44**   Hawkins classification

## Throwing Test

**Procedure and assessment:**  In the throwing test, the patient executes a rapid throwing motion against the examiner's resistance. This test can reveal anterior subluxation that occurs during the throwing motion.

## Leffert Test

**Procedure and assessment:** The Leffert test can be used to quantify a drawer phenomenon. Looking downward at the shoulder of the seated patient (craniocaudal view), the examiner displaces the humeral head anteriorly. The anterior displacement of the examiner's index finger in relation to the middle finger shows the degree of anterior translation of the humeral head.

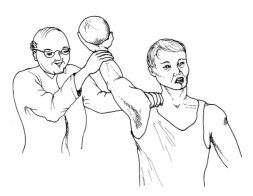

Fig. 2.**45**    Throwing test

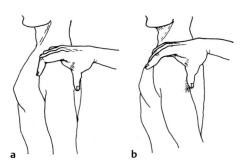

Fig. 2.**46a, b**    Leffert test:
**a** starting position,
**b** index finger displaced
    anteriorly

## Anterior and Posterior Load and Shift Test

**Procedure:**   The patient is seated. The examiner stands behind the patient. To evaluate the right shoulder, the examiner grasps the patient's shoulder with the left hand to stabilize the clavicle and superior margin of the scapula while using the right hand to move the humeral head anteriorly and posteriorly.

**Assessment:**   Significant anterior or posterior mobility of the humeral head suggests instability.

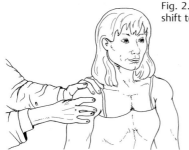

Fig. 2.**47**   Anterior and posterior lead and shift test

## Gerber–Ganz Anterior Drawer Test

**Procedure:**   The patient is supine with the affected shoulder positioned such that it projects slightly past the edge of the examining table. The affected shoulder is held in 80°–120° of abduction, 0°–20° of flexion, and 0°–30° of external rotation as loosely and without pain as possible. The examiner immobilizes the scapula with the left hand (with the index and middle fingers on the scapular spine and the thumb on the coracoid). With the right hand, the examiner tightly grasps the patient's proximal upper arm and pulls it anteriorly in a manner similar to the Lachman test for anterior instability in the knee.

**Assessment:**   The relative motion between the immobilized scapula and the anteriorly displaced humerus is a measure of anterior instability and can be classified in degrees.

Occasional audible clicking with or without pain can indicate an anterior labrum defect.

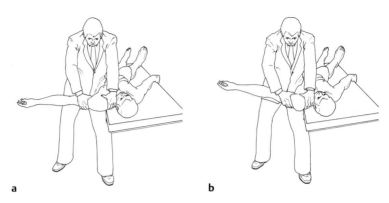

Fig. 2.**48a, b**   Gerber–Ganz anterior drawer test:
**a** starting position,
**b** dislocation maneuver

## Posterior Apprehension Test (Posterior Shift and Load Test)

**Procedure:**   With the patient supine, the examiner places one hand under the patient's scapula and grasps the elbow with the other. By pressing the abducted, horizontally flexed, and internally rotated arm posteriorly, the examiner attempts to provoke posterior subluxation of the humeral head.

**Assessment:**   Sufficient laxity in the capsular ligaments will allow posterior subluxation or even dislocation of the humeral head with associated pain.

Maintaining the axial pressure on the humeral head increasingly abducts and retracts the arm. The previously subluxated or dislocated humeral head can be reduced again with a readily palpable and audible click. (Caution: This test involves a certain risk of acute dislocation.)

## Gerber–Ganz Posterior Drawer Test

**Procedure:**   The patient is supine. Guiding the humeral head with one hand (with the thumb on the anterior humeral head and the fingers on the scapular spine, posterior humeral head, and scapular spine and posterior glenoid if necessary), with the other hand the examiner holds the patient's arm in 90° of flexion at about 20°–30° of horizontal extension.

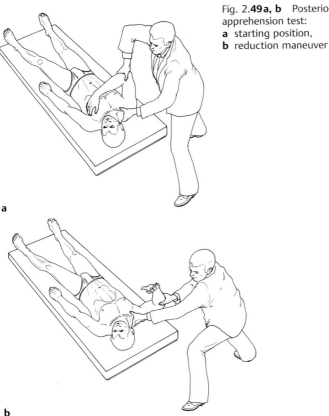

Fig. 2.**49a, b**  Posterior apprehension test:
**a** starting position,
**b** reduction maneuver

The examiner exerts pressure on the anterior humeral head with the thumb while simultaneously holding the arm in horizontal flexion and applying axial posterior compression in slight internal rotation.

**Assessment:**  Where there is sufficient laxity in the capsular ligaments, this test will provoke a posterior drawer (subluxation or dislocation of the humeral head). Horizontal extension, slight external rotation of the arm, and additional posteroanterior pressure applied by the finger to the posterior aspect of the humeral head will suffice to reduce the humeral head. The snap that accompanies reduction must be carefully distinguished from anterior subluxation. The important thing is to

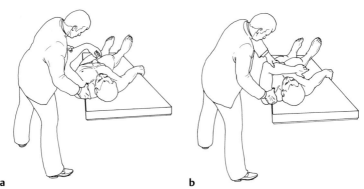

Fig. 2.**50a, b**   Gerber–Ganz posterior drawer test:
**a** starting position,
**b** dislocation maneuver

assess the motion of the humeral head relative to the glenoid fossa by placing the index finger posteriorly around the glenoid and pressing the humeral head in an anteroposterior direction with the thumb.

The examination may also be performed with the patient seated. With the patient in a relaxed posture bending slightly forward with the arm hanging alongside the trunk, the examiner places his or her thumb on the patient's scapular spine or posterior glenoid and grasps the humeral head anteriorly. Applying rotation and pressure with the fingers will provoke posterior subluxation of the head where there is sufficient laxity in the capsular ligaments.

In posterior instability, the humeral head can be posteriorly displaced by one-half its diameter.

### Posterior Apprehension Test with the Patient Standing

**Procedure:**   The patient is standing. The examiner abducts the affected arm between 90° and 110° at the shoulder and flexes it horizontally about 20°–30°. The examiner's other hand immobilizes the scapula from above; the examiner's fingers grasp the scapular spine and the humeral head while the thumb rests on the anterior aspect slightly lateral to the coracoid process.

**Assessment:**   With slowly increasing horizontal flexion, the posterior thrust along the longitudinal axis of the humerus leads to posterior

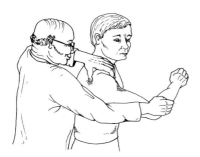 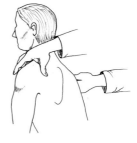

Fig. 2.**51**   Posterior apprehension test    Fig. 2.**52**   Fukuda test

subluxation in the glenohumeral joint. Both the thumb lateral to the coracoid process and the fingers can detect the translation of the humeral head. Occasionally, the slightly prominent humeral head will be visible beneath the acromion. Extending the arm by 20°–30° in the same horizontal plane will lead to palpable reduction of the humeral head.

## Fukuda Test

**Procedure and assessment:**   The Fukuda test elicits a passive posterior drawer sign. The patient is seated with the examiner's thumbs resting on both the patient's scapular spines. The examiner's other fingers rest anterior to the humeral head and exert posterior pressure to trigger a posterior drawer. This is usually done on both shoulders at the same time to compare the two sides.

## Sulcus Sign

Tests for multidirectional instability.

**Procedure:**   The patient is seated or standing. With one hand, the examiner stabilizes the patient's contralateral shoulder while exerting a distal pull on the patient's relaxed affected arm with the other hand. This is best done by grasping the patient's am at the elbow with the elbow slightly flexed.

**Assessment:**   Instability with distal displacement of the humeral head creates an obvious indentation (sulcus sign) inferior to the acromion.

The test can also be performed so that the examiner supports the patient's 90°-abducted arm. Applying pressure to the proximal third of

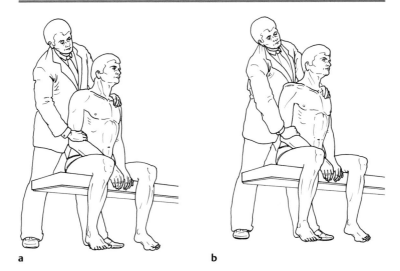

**a**                                              **b**

Fig. 2.**53a, b**   Sulcus sign:
**a** starting position,
**b** sulcus sign with distal distraction of the arm

the upper arm from above can then provoke distal subluxation of the humeral head. This will create a significant step-off beneath the acromion.

Aside from testing for the sulcus sign in the neutral position, it is recommended to perform the test with the arm externally and internally rotated as well. Increased inferior translation in external rotation suggests elongation of the rotator interval. A positive sulcus sign that occurs with the arm in internal rotation demonstrates laxity of the posterior capsular structures. Hyperlaxity in an inferior capsular ligament rupture can be demonstrated with the Gagey hyperabduction test. The examiner stands behind the patient and immobilizes the scapula with one hand. Achieving purely glenohumeral abduction over 105° suggests hyperlaxity of the inferior glenohumeral ligament in particular.

The sulcus sign may be graded by measuring from the inferior margin of the acromion to the humeral head. The typical system classifies a sulcus as grade I (< 1.5 cm), grade II (1.5–2.0 cm), or grade III (> 2 cm). A high-grade sulcus sign (grade III) is a sign of multidirectional instability.

## Rowe Test

**Procedure:** The patient stands and bends forward slightly with the arm relaxed. To examine the right shoulder, the examiner grasps the patient's shoulder with the left hand and with the right hand passively moves the patient's arm slightly anteriorly and inferiorly. The examiner then pulls the arms down slightly.

**Assessment:** To test for anterior instability the humeral head is pushed anteriorly with the thumb while the arm is extended 20°–30° from the vertical position. To test for posterior instability the humeral head is pushed posteriorly with the index and middle fingers while the arm is flexed 20°–30° from the vertical position. For inferior instability more traction is applied to the arm and the sulcus sign is evident.

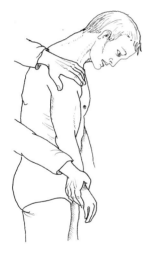

Fig. 2.**54**    Rowe test

# 3   Elbow

Because of its complexity, examination of the elbow and assessment of specific conditions can be difficult. Referred symptoms from other conditions with their origin in other areas like the cervical spine and shoulder have to be differentiated from local conditions. Initial important information can be gained from inspection. If the arm is held in flexion or if complex tasks like dressing and undressing cannot be performed adequately this can suggest various possible diagnoses (e. g., osteoarthritis or tendinitis).

Joint swelling is often most evident in the triangular space between radial head, olecranon, and laterale epicondyle (e. g., subcutaneous bursitis of the olecranon).

Axial deviation of the arm is a common cause of elbow problems (posttraumatic, congenital, dysplasias, etc.).

In arthritis, crepitation may be felt and heard at examination. The patient might describe locking of the elbow in the presence of free intraarticular bodies.

Injury to the collateral ligaments leads to instability of the joint. Epicondylitis is one of the most common reasons for complaints about and symptoms in the area of the elbow.

Pain felt along extensor tendons (tennis elbow or lateral epicondylitis) or flexor tendons (golfer's elbow or medial epicondylitis) is the result of repeated microtrauma to the tendon, leading to disruption and degeneration of the tendon's internal structure (tendinitis).

One common elbow condition around the elbow is bicipital tendinitis; the biceps can only be stretched to their full length by combining shoulder extension to its full length, elbow extension, and forearm pronation.

Strength is an important element of the physical examination, as adequate strength is a prerequisite to many functional activities. A quick scan of strength is sometimes performed using manual muscle tests (MMT) that are graded 0–5.

It has been shown that a muscle can produce a grade 5 level of strength using only 10% of the motor units.

For this reason, manual muscle testing is most useful in identification of disruption in motor nerve function that causes profound loss of strength arising from either compression neuropathy or acute nerve trauma.

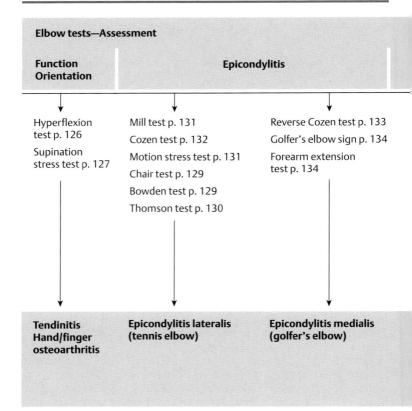

**Elbow tests—Assessment**

| **Function Orientation** | **Epicondylitis** | |
|---|---|---|

Hyperflexion test p. 126

Supination stress test p. 127

Mill test p. 131
Cozen test p. 132
Motion stress test p. 131
Chair test p. 129
Bowden test p. 129
Thomson test p. 130

Reverse Cozen test p. 133
Golfer's elbow sign p. 134
Forearm extension test p. 134

**Tendinitis Hand/finger osteoarthritis**

**Epicondylitis lateralis (tennis elbow)**

**Epicondylitis medialis (golfer's elbow)**

Fig. 3.**2**  Elbow tests

Table 3.**1**  Assessment of muscle strength

| Grade | Assessment | Description |
|---|---|---|
| 5 | Normal | Full range of motion against strong resistance |
| 4 | Good | Full range of motion against light resistance |
| 3 | Weak | Full range of motion against gravity |
| 2 | Very weak | Full range of motion without gravity |
| 1 | Slight | Visible and palpable activity, incomplete range of motion |
| 0 | Zero | Complete paralysis, no contraction |

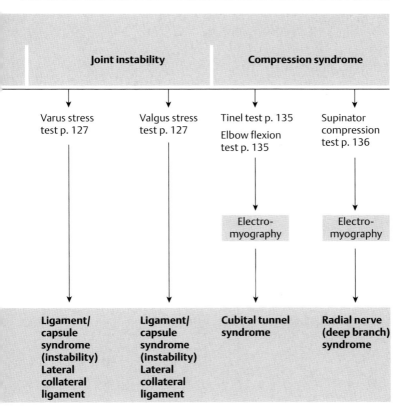

| Joint instability | | Compression syndrome | |
|---|---|---|---|
| Varus stress test p. 127 | Valgus stress test p. 127 | Tinel test p. 135<br><br>Elbow flexion test p. 135 | Supinator compression test p. 136 |
| | | Electro-myography | Electro-myography |
| **Ligament/ capsule syndrome (instability) Lateral collateral ligament** | **Ligament/ capsule syndrome (instability) Lateral collateral ligament** | **Cubital tunnel syndrome** | **Radial nerve (deep branch) syndrome** |

# ■ Range of Motion of the Elbow (Neutral-Zero Method)

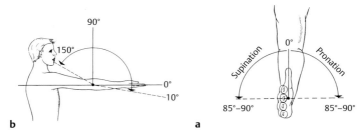

Fig. 3.**1a, b**
**a** Flexion and extension,
**b** pronation and supination of the forearm

# ■ Function Tests

This section describes a series of function tests that will indicate specific lesions in the region of the elbow. Those that provide the most diagnostic information are presented below. They have been divided into four groups based on the particular anatomic structure being tested.

1. General orientation tests
2. Stability tests
3. Epicondylitis tests
4. Compression syndrome tests

# ■ Orientation Tests

### Hyperflexion Test

Indicates the presence of an elbow disorder.

**Procedure:**   The patient is seated. The examiner grasps the patient's wrist and maximally flexes the elbow, carefully noting any restricted motion and the location of any pain.

**Assessment:**   Increased or restricted mobility in the joint coupled with pain is a sign of joint damage, muscle contracture, tendinitis, or a sprain.

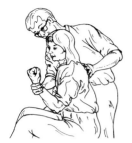

Fig. 3.**3a** Hyperflexion test

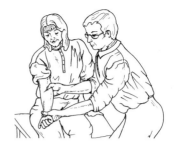

Fig. 3.**3b** Supination stress test

## Supination Stress Test

For diagnostic assessment of an elbow disorder.

**Procedure:** The patient is seated. The examiner grasps the patient's forearm with one hand while holding the medial aspect of the elbow with the other. From this position, the examiner forcibly and abruptly supinates the forearm.

**Assessment:** This test evaluates the integrity of the elbow including the bony and ligamentous structures. Pain or restricted motion suggests joint dysfunction requiring further examination.

## ■ Stability Tests

### Ligamentous Instability

The examiner applies force to the elbow joint repeatedly with increasing pressure while noting any alteration in pain or range of motion. If excessive laxity or a soft endpoint is found this indicates ligamentous injury or joint instability.

The examiner should note any alteration in laxity, mobility, or pain that may be present compared to the uninvolved elbow.

### Ligamentous Instability Test

Evaluation of varus and valgus instability of the elbow joint.

The patient sits with the elbow slightly flexed. The examiner stabilizes the upper arm medially with one hand while, with the other hand,

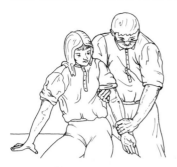

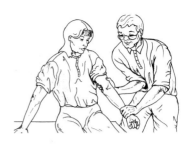

Fig. 3.**4**   Varus stress test                Fig. 3.**5**   Valgus stress test

adducting the patient's forearm in the elbow joint. This creates varus stress to the lateral collateral ligament (varus instability).

An abduction or valgus force to the distal forearm is then applied in a similar fashion to test the medial collateral ligament (valgus instability).

### Posterolateral Rotary Instability Elbow Test (Pivot Shift Test)

Posterolateral elbow instability is the most common pattern of elbow instability in which there is displacement of the ulna (accompanied by the radius) in the elbow.

**Procedure:** The patient is supine. The examiner stands at the head of the patient and grasps the patient's wrist and extended elbow. A mild supination force is applied to the forearm at the wrist. The patient's elbow is then flexed while a valgus stress and compression is applied to the elbow.

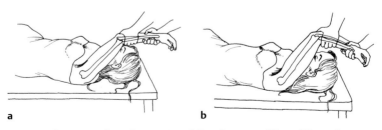

a                                              b

Fig. 3.**6a, b**   Posterolateral rotary instability elbow test (Pivot shift test):
**a** the elbow is flexed between 20° and 30° (subluxation),
**b** flexing the elbow from 40° to 70° (reduction)

**Assessment:**   If posterolateral instability is present, the patient will be apprehensive when the elbow is being flexed (between 20° and 30°). The patient expects the elbow to dislocate posterolaterally. If the examiner continues flexing the elbow to 40°–70°, there is a sudden reduction of the joint which can be palpated and observed.

## ■ Epicondylitis Tests

### Chair Test

Indicates lateral epicondylitis.

**Procedure:**   The patient is requested to lift a chair. The arm should be extended with the forearm pronated.

**Assessment:**   Occurrence of or increase in pain over the lateral epicondyle and in the extensor tendon origins in the forearm indicates epicondylitis.

### Bowden Test

Indicates tennis elbow (lateral epicondylitis).

**Procedure:**   The patient is requested to squeeze together a blood-pressure measuring cuff inflated to about 30 mmHg (about 4.0 kPa)

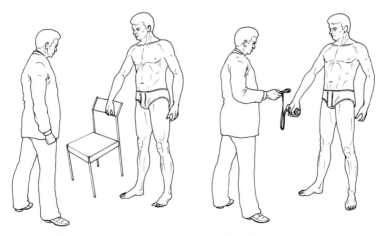

Fig. 3.**7**   Chair test                    Fig. 3.**8**   Bowden test

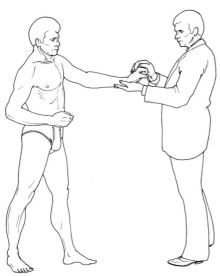

Fig. 3.**9**    Thomson test

held in his or her hand, or, by squeezing the cuff, to maintain a pressure specified by the examiner.

**Assessment:**   Occurrence of or increase in pain over the lateral epicondyle and in the extensor tendon origins in the forearm indicates epicondylitis.

### Thomson Test

Indicates lateral epicondylitis.

**Procedure:**   The patient is requested to make a fist and extend the elbow with the hand in slight dorsiflexion. The examiner immobilizes the dorsal wrist with one hand and grasps the fist with the other hand. The patient is then requested to further extend the fist against the examiner's resistance, or the examiner attempts to press the dorsiflexed fist into flexion against the patient's resistance.

**Assessment:**   Severe pain over the lateral epicondyle and in the lateral extensor compartment strongly suggests lateral epicondylitis.

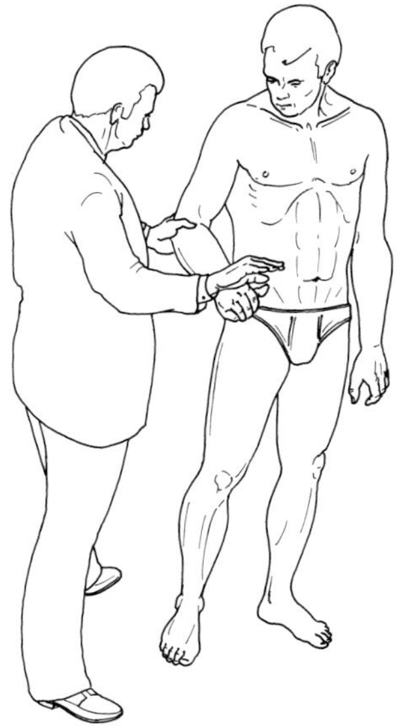

Fig. 3.**10**   Mill test

## Mill Test

Indicates lateral epicondylitis.

**Procedure:**   The patient is standing. The arm is slightly pronated with the wrist slightly dorsiflexed and the elbow flexed. With one hand, the examiner grasps the patient's elbow while the other rests on the lateral aspect of the distal forearm or grasps the forearm. The patient is then requested to supinate the forearm against the resistance of the examiner's hand.

**Assessment:**   Pain over the lateral epicondyle and/or in the lateral extensors suggests epicondylitis.

## Motion Stress Test

Indicates lateral epicondylitis.

**Procedure:**   The patient is seated. The examiner palpates the lateral epicondyle while the patient flexes the elbow, pronates the forearm, and then extends the elbow again in a continuous motion.

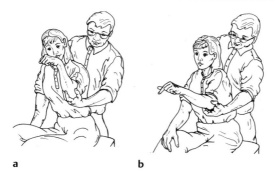

Fig. 3.**11a, b**
Motion stress test:
**a** starting position,
**b** extension and
pronation

a                              b

**Assessment:**   Pronation and wrist flexion place great stresses on the
tendons of the forearm musculature that arise from the lateral epicondyle. Occurrence of pain in the lateral epicondyle and/or lateral extensor
musculature with these motions suggests epicondylitis. However, pain
and paresthesia can also occur as a result of compression of the median
nerve because in this maneuver the action of the pronators can compress the nerve.

### Cozen Test

Indicates lateral epicondylitis.

**Procedure:**   The patient is seated for the examination. The examiner
immobilizes the elbow with one hand while the other hand lies flat on
the dorsum of the patient's fist. The patient is then requested to dorsi-

Fig. 3.**12**   Cozen test

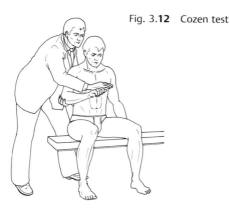

flex the wrist against the resistance of the examiner's hand. Alternatively, the examiner may attempt to press the fist, which the patient holds with the wrist firmly extended, into flexion against the patient's resistance.

**Assessment:** Localized pain in the lateral epicondyle of the humerus or pain in the lateral extensor compartment suggests epicondylitis.

### Reverse Cozen Test

Indicates medial epicondylitis.

**Procedure:** The patient is seated. The examiner palpates the medial epicondyle with one hand while the other hand rests on the wrist of the patient's supinated forearm. The patient attempts to flex the extended hand against the resistance of the examiner's hand on the wrist.

**Assessment:** The flexors of the forearm and hand and the pronator teres have their origins on the medial epicondyle. Acute, stabbing pain over the medial epicondyle suggests medial epicondylitis.

With this test, it is particularly important to stabilize the elbow. Otherwise, a forcible avoidance movement or pronation could exacerbate a compression syndrome in the pronator musculature (pronator compartment syndrome).

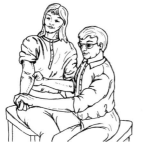
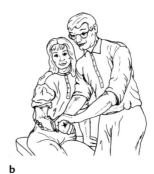
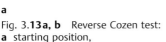

**a**          **b**

Fig. 3.**13a, b**   Reverse Cozen test:
**a** starting position,
**b** flexion in the wrist against the resistance of the examiner's hand

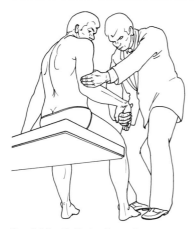

Fig. 3.**14**   Golfer's elbow sign

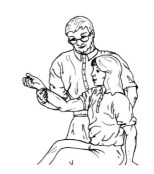

Fig. 3.**15**   Forearm extension test

### Golfer's Elbow Sign

Indicates medial epicondylitis.

**Procedure:**   The patient flexes the elbow and hand. The examiner grasps the patient's hand and immobilizes the patient's upper arm with the other hand. The patient is then requested to extend the elbow against the resistance of the examiner's hand.

**Assessment:**   Pain over the medial epicondyle suggests epicondylar pathology (golfer's elbow).

### Forearm Extension Test

Indicates medial epicondylitis.

**Procedure:**   The seated patient flexes the elbow and holds the forearm in supination while the examiner grasps the patient's distal forearm. The patient then attempts to extend the elbow against the resistance of the examiner's hand.

**Assessment:**   Pain over the medial epicondyle and over the origins of the forearm flexors suggests epicondylar pathology.

# ■ Compression Syndrome Tests

### Tinel Test

Sign of cubital tunnel syndrome.

**Procedure:** The patient is seated. The examiner grasps the patient's arms and gently taps on the groove for the ulnar nerve with a reflex hammer.

**Assessment:** The ulnar nerve courses through a bony groove posterior to the medial epicondyle. Because of its relatively superficial position, compression injuries are common. Injury, traction, inflammation, scarring, or chronic compression are the most common causes of damage to the ulnar nerve. Pain elicited by gently tapping the groove for the ulnar nerve suggests chronic compression neuropathy.

With this test, care should be taken not to tap the nerve too hard because a forceful tap will cause pain even in a normal nerve. Note, too, that repeated tapping can injure the nerve.

### Elbow Flexion Test

Sign of cubital tunnel syndrome.

**Procedure:** The patient is seated. The elbow is maximally flexed with the wrist flexed as well. The patient is requested to maintain this position for five minutes.

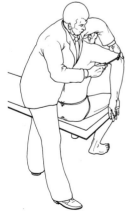

Fig. 3.**16** Tinel test

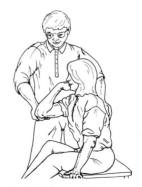

Fig. 3.**17** Elbow flexion test

**Assessment:**   The ulnar nerve passes through the cubital tunnel, which is formed by the ulnar collateral ligaments and the flexor carpi ulnaris. Maximum traction is applied to the ulnar nerve in the position described above.

Occurrence of paresthesia along the course of the nerve suggests compressive neuropathy. If the test is positive, the diagnosis should be confirmed by electromyography or nerve conduction velocity measurement.

### Supinator Compression Test

Indicates damage to the deep branch of the radial nerve.

**Procedure:**   The patient is seated. With one hand, the examiner palpates the groove lateral to the extensor carpi radialis distal to the lateral epicondyle. The examiner's other hand resists the patient's active pronation and supination.

**Assessment:**   Constant pain in the muscle groove or pain in the proximal lateral forearm that increases with pronation and supination suggests compression of the deep branch of the radial nerve in the supinator (the deep branch of the radial nerve penetrates this muscle).

The point of tenderness lies farther anterior than the point at which pain is felt in typical lateral epicondylitis. The compression neuropathy of the nerve can be caused by proliferation of connective tissue in the muscle, a radial head fracture, or a soft tissue tumor. Weakened or absent extension in the metacarpophalangeal joints of the fingers other than the thumb indicates paralysis of the extensor digitorum supplied by the deep branch of the radial nerve.

Fig. 3.**18**   Supinator compression test

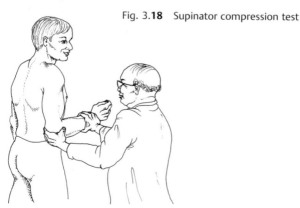

# 4 Wrist, Hand, and Fingers

Injuries to and lesions of the hand play a significant role in everyday life and in sports.

Examination of the hand requires good knowledge of the functional anatomy and begins with inspection to detect possible defects and position anomalies. With the hand at rest in a passive position, the wrist is in a neutral position between flexion and extension and the fingers are in slight flexion (the finger flexors are about four times as strong as the finger extensors).

Joint inflammation causes circumscribed swelling over the respective joint, and tenosynovitis manifests itself as swelling and erythema in the skin along the course of the tendon. Swelling of the distal interphalangeal joints with a painful flexion contracture (Heberden nodes) often occurs in postmenopausal women. Chronic inflammatory disorders (rheumatoid arthritis) often first manifest themselves in the metacarpophalangeal and proximal interphalangeal joints.

Ganglia arising from the tendons, tendon sheath, or synovial tissue may be the cause of swelling. Nerve palsy leads to contractures. For example, radial nerve palsy leads to a limp wrist. Median nerve palsy leads to deformity resembling an ape's hand. Ulnar nerve palsy leads to a claw hand deformity in which the proximal phalanges are extended and the middle and distal phalanges are flexed.

When palpating the wrist and hand, the examiner notes the texture and quality of the skin, muscles, and tendon sheaths; evaluates swelling, inflammation, and tumors; and determines the exact localization of pain.

Passive range of motion testing can detect restricted motion (due to osteoarthritis) and instability. Painful disorders of the tendon sheaths can be associated with crepitation along the course of the tendon in both active and passive motion.

Neurologic changes such as muscle atrophy, usually caused by compression neuropathies, exhibit characteristic losses of function that can be evaluated by specific functional tests.

## ■ Range of Motion in the Hand (Neutral-Zero Method)

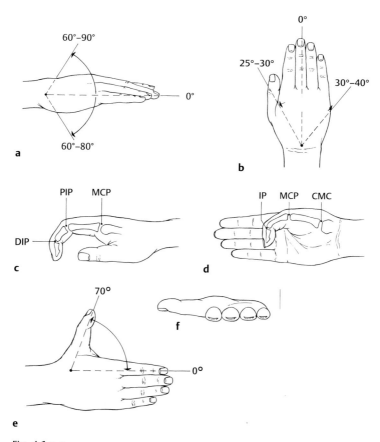

Fig. 4.**1a–s**
**a**      Flexion and extension of the wrist including the intercarpal joint.
**b**      Radial and ulnar deviation of the hand.
**c, d**  Designations of the joints of the fingers (**c**) and thumb (**d**):
         *DIP* = distal interphalangeal joint, *PIP* = proximal interphalangeal joint,
         *MCP* = metacarpophalangeal joint, *IP* = interphalangeal joint (of the thumb),
         *CMC* = carpometacarpal joint
**e, f**  Abduction and adduction to the plane of the palm.

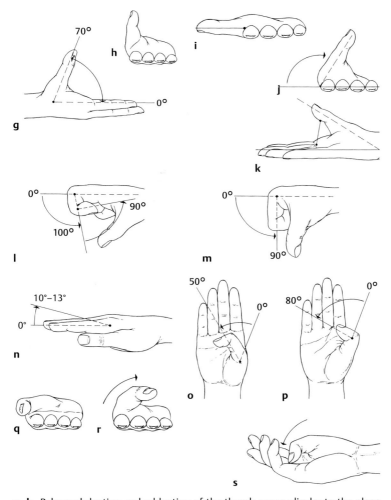

g, h  Palmar abduction and adduction of the thumb perpendicular to the plane of the palm.

i–k  Circumduction of the extended thumb.

l, m  Flexion of the finger joints: DIP and PIP joints (l) and MCP joint (m).

n  Hyperextension of the MCP joint.

o, p  Flexion of the thumb joints: the MCP $_1$ joint (o) and the IP joint (p).

q–s  Opposition of the thumb: starting position (q), during motion (r), and in opposition position (s)

**Hand tests—Assessment**

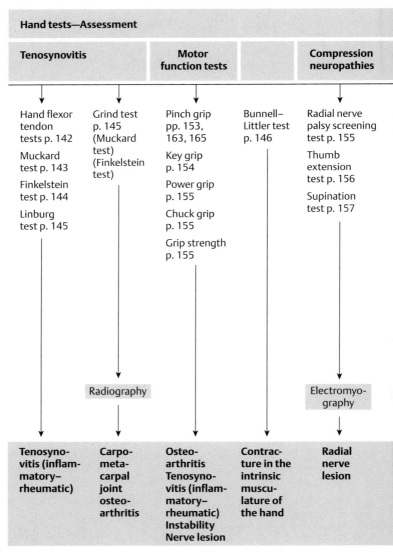

| Tenosynovitis | | Motor function tests | | Compression neuropathies |
|---|---|---|---|---|
| Hand flexor tendon tests p. 142 | Grind test p. 145 (Muckard test) (Finkelstein test) | Pinch grip pp. 153, 163, 165 | Bunnell–Littler test p. 146 | Radial nerve palsy screening test p. 155 |
| Muckard test p. 143 | | Key grip p. 154 | | Thumb extension test p. 156 |
| Finkelstein test p. 144 | | Power grip p. 155 | | Supination test p. 157 |
| Linburg test p. 145 | | Chuck grip p. 155 | | |
| | | Grip strength p. 155 | | |
| | Radiography | | | Electromyography |
| Tenosynovitis (inflammatory–rheumatic) | Carpometacarpal joint osteoarthritis | Osteoarthritis Tenosynovitis (inflammatory–rheumatic) Instability Nerve lesion | Contracture in the intrinsic musculature of the hand | Radial nerve lesion |

Fig. 4.**2** Hand, wrist, and finger tests

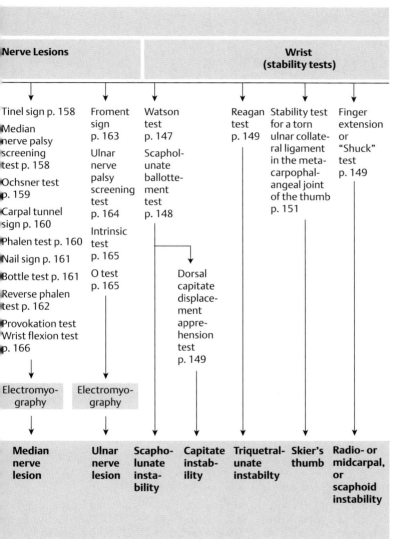

| Nerve Lesions | | | Wrist (stability tests) | | |
|---|---|---|---|---|---|

Tinel sign p. 158

Median nerve palsy screening test p. 158

Ochsner test p. 159

Carpal tunnel sign p. 160

Phalen test p. 160

Nail sign p. 161

Bottle test p. 161

Reverse phalen test p. 162

Provokation test Wrist flexion test p. 166

↓

Electromyography

---

Froment sign p. 163

Ulnar nerve palsy screening test p. 164

Intrinsic test p. 165

O test p. 165

↓

Electromyography

---

Watson test p. 147

Scapholunate ballottement test p. 148

↓

Dorsal capitate displacement apprehension test p. 149

---

Reagan test p. 149

---

Stability test for a torn ulnar collateral ligament in the metacarpophalangeal joint of the thumb p. 151

---

Finger extension or "Shuck" test p. 149

---

**Median nerve lesion**

**Ulnar nerve lesion**

**Scapholunate instability**

**Capitate instability**

**Triquetralunate instabilty**

**Skier's thumb**

**Radio- or midcarpal, or scaphoid instability**

## ■ Function Tests

### Tests of the Flexor Tendons of the Hand

#### *Flexor Digitorum Profundus*

**Procedure:**  The examiner places two fingers (index and middle fingers) on the volar aspect of the patient's affected finger so that the finger remains extended in the proximal interphalangeal joint. The patient is then asked to flex only the distal interphalangeal joint of the finger. This examination is repeated for each finger separately.

**Assessment:**  The flexor digitorum profundus belongs the deep layer of flexors in the forearm. Its tendons insert into the bases of all of the proximal phalanges of the fingers.

Inability to flex the distal interphalangeal joint is a sign of a torn tendon; painful flexion suggests tenosynovitis.

Differential diagnosis should exclude osteoarthritis of the distal interphalangeal joint (Heberden nodes) with a painful flexion contracture.

#### *Flexor Digitorum Superficialis*

**Procedure:**  The patient is asked to flex the proximal interphalangeal joint of the affected finger while the examiner holds the other fingers in extension to neutralize the effect of the flexor digitorum profundus tendon. The flexor digitorum profundus tendons of the three ulnar fingers share a common muscle belly. Therefore, unrestricted flexion of one finger with the others immobilized in extension requires an intact flexor digitorum superficialis tendon. This examination is performed for each finger separately.

**Assessment:**  The flexor digitorum superficialis is a broad strong muscle whose tendons insert into the middle phalanges of the fingers.

Wherever the patient can flex the proximal interphalangeal joint of a finger, the flexor digitorum superficialis tendon is intact. Flexion will not be possible where injuries to the tendon are present. Pain suggests tenosynovitis.

#### *Flexor Pollicis Longus and Extensor Pollicis Longus*

**Procedure:**  The examiner grasps the patient's thumb and immobilizes the metacarpophalangeal joint. Then the patient is asked to flex and extend the phalanx of the thumb. The flexor pollicis longus lies in the deep layer of the flexor muscles; its tendon inserts into the base of the distal phalanx of the thumb.

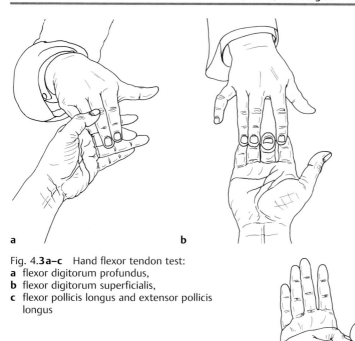

Fig. 4.**3a–c**   Hand flexor tendon test:
**a** flexor digitorum profundus,
**b** flexor digitorum superficialis,
**c** flexor pollicis longus and extensor pollicis longus

**Assessment:**   Impaired flexion and extension in the interphalangeal joint of the thumb suggest injury (torn tendon) or disease (tenosynovitis) of the respective tendon.

### Muckard Test

For diagnosis of acute or chronic tenosynovitis of the abductor pollicis longus and extensor pollicis brevis tendons (stenosing tenosynovitis or de Quervain's disease).

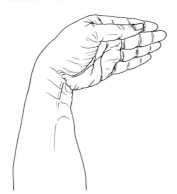

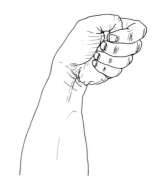

Fig. 4.**4**   Muckard test          Fig. 4.**5**   Finkelstein test

**Procedure:**   The patient "tilts" the hand into ulnar deviation at the wrist with the fingers extended and the thumb adducted.

**Assessment:**   Severe pain in the radial styloid radiating into the thumb and forearm suggests tenosynovitis of the abductor pollicis longus and extensor pollicis brevis tendons.

Swelling and tenderness to palpation over the first dorsal compartment will usually be present as well. Abduction of the thumb against resistance is painful.

Tenosynovitis is the result of inflammation of the synovial tissue, which is often caused by overuse or inflammatory disorders. However, blunt trauma can also lead to these disorders.

A differential diagnosis should exclude osteoarthritis of the carpometacarpal joint of the thumb or radial styloiditis.

### Finkelstein Test

Indicates stenosing tenosynovitis (de Quervain's disease).

**Procedure:**   With the thumb flexed and the other fingers flexed around it, the wrist is moved into ulnar deviation either actively or passively by the examiner.

**Assessment:**   Pain and crepitation above the radial styloid suggest nonspecific tenosynovitis of the abductor pollicis longus and the extensor pollicis brevis (see Muckard test for etiology).

It is important to differentiate stenosing tenosynovitis (de Quervain's disease) from osteoarthritis in the carpometacarpal joint of the thumb.

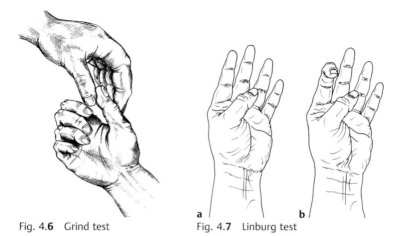

Fig. 4.**6**   Grind test          Fig. 4.**7**   Linburg test

Specific examination of the carpometacarpal joint of the thumb and a radiograph will allow a quick differential diagnosis.

The test should also be performed on both sides for comparison.

### Grind Test

Assessment of osteoarthritis in the carpometacarpal joint of the thumb.

**Procedure:**   The examiner grasps the painful thumb and performs grinding motions while compressing the thumb along its longitudinal axis.

**Assessment:**   Pain reported in the carpometacarpal joint of the thumb is usually due to osteoarthritis in the joint (differential diagnosis includes a Bennet or Rolando fracture). Tenderness to palpation and painful instability are additional signs of wear in the joint. The patient will typically also complain of pain in the carpometacarpal joint of the thumb when opposing the thumb against the resistance of the examiner's hand.

### Linburg Test

Indicates congenital malformation of the flexor pollicis longus and flexor digitorum profundus tendons.

**Procedure:**   The patient is asked to bring the thumb against the palm of the hand in a combined flexion and adduction motion with the fingers extended.

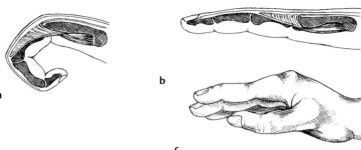

Fig. 4.**8a–c**   Bunnell–Littler test:
**a** active and passive flexion of all finger joints is possible (first part),
**b** metacarpophalangeal joint is immobilized in extension; flexion of the middle and distal phalangeal joints is not possible (second part),
**c** intrinsic plus deformity

**Assessment:**   In the presence of a congenital ligamentous connection between the flexor pollicis longus tendon and flexor digitorum profundus tendon of the index finger, this combined thumb motion will produce flexion in the distal interphalangeal joint of the index finger. This is an anomalous tendon condition seen in 10% to 15% of hands.

### Bunnell–Littler Test

Assessment of an ischemic contracture in the intrinsic musculature of the hand.

**Procedure:**   The patient's hand is extended. In the first part of the test, the examiner evaluates passive and active flexion in all three joints of a finger. In the second part of the test, the examiner immobilizes the metacarpophalangeal joint in extension and again evaluates flexion in the middle and distal interphalangeal joints of the finger.

**Assessment:**   In the presence of an ischemic contracture of the intrinsic muscles of the hand, the patient will be unable to actively or passively flex or extend the middle or distal interphalangeal joint when the metacarpophalangeal joint is passively immobilized in extension. This is due to shortening of the interossei. With the wrist actively or passively flexed, active flexion of the middle and distal interphalangeal joints is possible. Usually the contracture will affect several fingers. The test allows one to distinguish an ischemic contracture from other articular changes such as joint stiffness, tendon adhesions, and tenosynovitis.

Increased pressure in the fascial compartments of the hand produces a typical deformity with slight flexion in the metacarpophalangeal

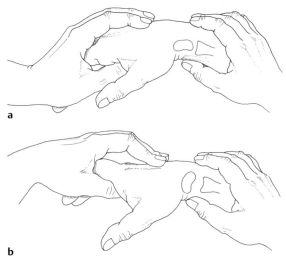

**b**
Fig. 4.**9a, b** Watson test (scaphoid shift test):
**a** wrist in radial deviation; immobilization of the scaphoid in extension,
**b** wrist placed in ulnar deviation

joints, extension in the middle and distal interphalangeal joints, intensification of the transverse arch of the hand, and adduction of the thumb (intrinsic plus deformity).

### Watson Test (Scaphoid Shift Test)

Tests wrist stability.

**Procedure:** The examiner takes the patient's wrist with one hand and positions it in full ulnar deviation and slight extension while feeling for the metacarpals.

Then the examiner presses with the thumb of the other hand and against the distal pole of the scaphoid on the palmar side to prevent it from moving "into" the palm while the fingers apply counter pressure to the back of the forearm. With the first hand the examiner radially deviates and slightly flexes the patient's hand while maintaining pressure on the scaphoid. This creates a subluxation stress to the possibly unstable scaphoid bone.

**Assessment:** The test is positive (scaphoid and lunate are unstable) when the dorsal pole of the scaphoid subluxates or shifts beyond the dorsal rim of the radius and the patient complains of pain.

If the scaphoid subluxates with the thumb pressure, when the thumb is removed the scaphoid usually returns back to its normal position with a "thunk." If the ligamentous tissues are intact, the scaphoid will mostly move forward pushing the thumb in the same direction.

### Scapholunate Ballottement Test

Tests wrist stability.

**Procedure:**  The examiner holds the scaphoid and lunate tightly between the thumb and index finger of both hands while moving them relative to each other in a dorsal and volar direction, respectively.

**Assessment:**  Instability is present where the resistance of the scapholunate ligament complex to these shear forces is reduced. Painful shear motion indicates a ligament injury. Scapholunate instability occurs as a result of a fall on the thumb with the forearm pronated and the wrist extended and in ulnar deviation, or as the result of an impact in ball sports. This causes a tear in the ligaments between the scaphoid and lunate. Chronic scapholunate instability can also occur without trauma, for example secondary to removal of a ganglion or in degenerative disorders. Patients complain of severe tenderness to palpation and pain with motion in the proximal radial wrist, especially when supporting the body with the hands. They also report loss of strength and occasionally describe a snapping sound when moving the wrist into ulnar deviation.

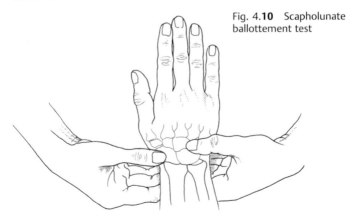

Fig. 4.**10**   Scapholunate ballottement test

### Reagan Test (Lunotriquetral Ballottement Test)

Evaluation of the integrity of the lunotriquetral ligament.

**Procedure:**   The examiner grasps the lunate between the thumb and forefinger with one hand and the triquetrum between the fingers of the other hand. The examiner then moves the lunatum up and down.

**Assessment:**   In a positive test, this shear motion is painful even if instability cannot always be demonstrated.

Triquetrolunate instability can result from trauma involving hyperpronation or hyperextension. Patients report pain in the wrist. Tenderness to palpation over the triquetrolunate joint and pain with motion can be provoked, but pronation and supination do not casue any pain. The injury does not necessarily involve loss of strength. Patients occasionally describe the instability as a clicking that occurs during wrist motion.

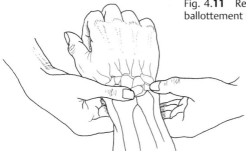

Fig. 4.**11**   Reagan test (triquetrolunate ballottement test)

### Finger Extension or "Shuck" Test

**Procedure:**   The examiner holds the sitting patient's wrist flexed and asks the patient to actively extend the fingers against resistance loading the radiocarpal joint.

**Assessment:**   Test is positive when pain occurs. Pain can indicate radiocarpal or midcarpal instability, scaphoid instability, inflammation, or Kienböck disease.

### Dorsal Capitate Displacement Apprehension Test

Determination of the stability of the capitate bone.

**Procedure:**   The examiner holds the forearm of the sitting patient with one hand. The thumb of the examiner's other hand is placed over the

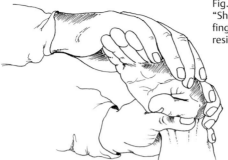

Fig. 4.**12**   Finger extension or "Shuck" test: wrist flexed and the fingers actively extend against resistance

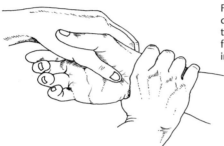

Fig. 4.**13**   Dorsal capitate displacement apprehension test: the examiner's thumb and long fingers hold the patients fingers in a neutral position

palmar aspect of the capitate while the examiner's fingers hold the patient's fingers in a neutral position and apply a counter pressure. The examiner then pushes the capitate posteriorly with the thumb.

**Assessment:**   The test is positive when the patient's symptoms can be reproduced, with apprehension or pain. A click or snap may also be heard when pressure is applied.

### Supination Lift Test

Testing for pathology of the triangular fibrocartilaginous complex (triangular cartilaginous disk).

**Procedure:**   The patient is sitting with the elbows flexed at 90° and forearms supine.

The patient is then asked to place the palms flat against the examiner's hands and to push up against the counter pressure of the examiner's hands.

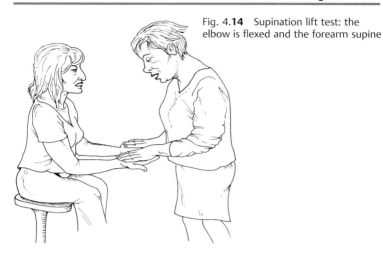

Fig. 4.**14**   Supination lift test: the elbow is flexed and the forearm supine

**Assessment:**   Localized pain on the ulnar side of the wrist and difficulty applying the force are positive indications for a dorsal triangular cartilaginous disk tear.

### Stability Test for a Torn Ulnar Collateral Ligament in the Metacarpophalangeal Joint of the Thumb

**Procedure:**   The patient flexes the metacarpophalangeal joint of the affected thumb 20°–30°. The examiner passively moves the thumb into radial deviation.

**Assessment:**   Where the thumb can be abducted, this suggests a tear in the ulnar collateral ligament of the metacarpophalangeal joint of the thumb. Known as gamekeeper's or skier's thumb, this injury is caused by forced radial deviation of the extended thumb in a fall on the hand. Stability is tested with the thumb flexed 20°–30°. This is done to minimize the action of the accessory collateral ligament, which, if intact, could mask the tear in the collateral ligament in extension. Where the joint can be opened in extension, one may assume that a complex injury to the capsular ligaments is present.

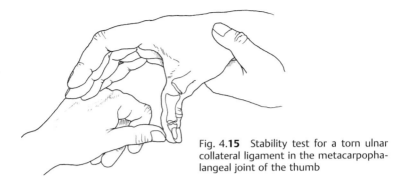

Fig. 4.**15**  Stability test for a torn ulnar collateral ligament in the metacarpophalangeal joint of the thumb

## Compression Neuropathies of the Nerves of the Arm

A number of compression neuropathies and entrapment syndromes can affect the nerves of the arm. Clinical tests can help differentiate between them.

### Pronator Teres Syndrome

The median nerve can become compressed between the humeral and ulnar heads of the pronator teres.

There are a number of possible causes for a pronator teres syndrome. These include external pressure on the forearm, hypertrophy of the pronator teres (muscle tremor), and direct trauma. Pain, a burning sensation, and sensory deficits in the hand are typical symptoms, as are weakness in thumb opposition and weakness in flexion in the thumb, index finger, and middle finger. Pronation against resistance exacerbates the symptoms.

### Compression Neuropathy of the Ulnar Nerve in Guyon's Canal

Guyon's canal is formed by the flexor retinaculum, pisohamate ligament, and palmar aponeurosis. The ulnar artery and nerve course through this passage.

Causes of compression of the ulnar nerve include acute and chronic trauma, such as chronic compression injury in bicyclists.

Sensory impairments in the ulnar aspect of the ring and little fingers and motor impairments in the hypothenar musculature are typical symptoms of this compression neuropathy.

### Carpal Tunnel Syndrome

Compression of the median nerve can occur in the carpal tunnel. Formed by the carpal bones and the flexor retinaculum, the carpal tunnel encloses all of the finger flexor tendons and the median nerve. Causes of carpal tunnel syndrome with stenosis of the tunnel include skeletal changes, bone tumors (ganglia), injuries, and tenosynovitis. Women between the ages of 50 and 60 are most commonly affected. Typical signs of compression include nighttime paresthesia and brachialgia, morning stiffness, and sensory and motor deficits in the region supplied by the median nerve (atrophy of the thenar musculature).

A differential diagnosis should consider cervical spinal cord and brachial plexus lesions, pronator teres syndrome, compression neuropathy in Guyon's canal, thoracic outlet syndrome, and interphalangeal osteoarthritis.

Electromyography and measurement of nerve conduction velocity by electroneurography are important studies in diagnosing carpal tunnel syndrome.

### Cubital Tunnel Syndrome

The ulnar nerve courses through a bony groove posterior to the medial epicondyle. Because of its relatively superficial position, compression injuries are common. Injury, traction, inflammation, scarring, or chronic compression are the most common causes of damage to the ulnar nerve.

Sensory deficits (numbness in the little finger) and motor deficits in the area supplied by the ulnar nerve are typical findings in the presence of a nerve lesion.

Electromyography and sensory electroneurography can determine the location of the compression neuropathy.

## Tests of Motor Function in the Hand

Demonstrate motor and sensory deficits in the presence of nerve lesions.

### Testing the Pinch Grip

**Procedure:** The patient is asked to pick up a small object between the thumb and the index finger.

**Assessment:** Satisfactory performance requires intact sensation. The patient should repeat the test with his or her eyes closed. Unimpaired function of the lumbricals and interossei is essential for this maneuver.

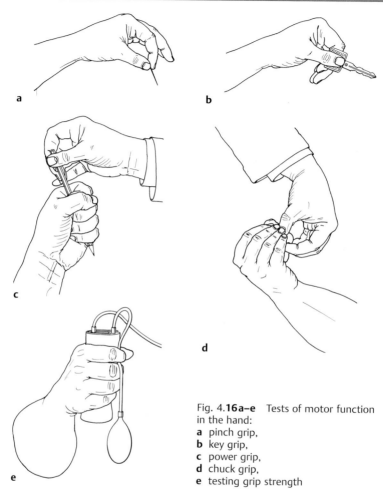

Fig. 4.**16a–e**   Tests of motor function in the hand:
**a** pinch grip,
**b** key grip,
**c** power grip,
**d** chuck grip,
**e** testing grip strength

### Testing the Key Grip

**Procedure:**   The patient is asked to hold a key between the thumb and the side of the index finger in the normal manner.

**Assessment:**   A sensory deficit on the radial aspect of the index finger, such as can occur in a radial nerve lesion, renders the key grip impossible.

### Testing the Power Grip

**Procedure:** The patient is asked to hold on to a pencil with the thumb and fingers while the examiner attempts to pull the pencil away.

Where finger flexion is restricted, the test is repeated using an object with a larger diameter.

**Assessment:** In the presence of injuries to the median or ulnar nerve, full finger flexion is not possible and strength is limited. The test will be positive in these cases.

### Testing the Chuck Grip

**Procedure:** The precision grip maneuver is evaluated by giving the patient a small ball and having him or her hold on to it.

**Assessment:** This maneuver tests the strength of adduction in the thumb and finger flexion and thus allows evaluation of the median and ulnar nerves to be assessed.

### Testing Grip Strength

**Procedure:** The examiner pumps a blood pressure cuff to 200 mmHg (about 26.7 kPa) and asks the patient to squeeze it together as tightly as possible.

**Assessment:** Patients with normal hand function should attain a value of 200 mmHg (about 26.7 kPa) or more. Note that the difference in strength between men and women must be taken into account, as must that between adults and children. This test should be performed with each hand for comparative evaluation.

### Radial Nerve Palsy Screening Test

Screening method for the assessment of radial nerve palsy.

**Procedure:** The patient is asked to extend his or her wrist with the elbow flexed 90°.

**Assessment:** In radial nerve palsy affecting the wrist extensors, the patient will be unable to extend the wrist. The hand will hang down in a deformity commonly known as a limp wrist. In a second stage of the test, the patient is asked to abduct the thumb. In radial nerve palsy, the patient will be unable to abduct the thumb because of the paralysis of the abductor pollicis longus.

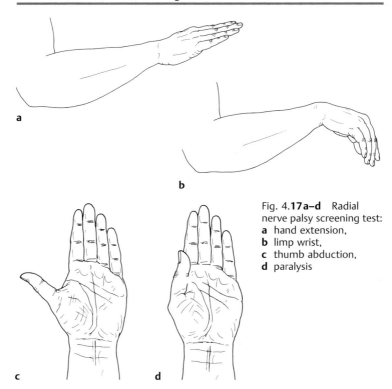

Fig. 4.**17a–d**   Radial nerve palsy screening test:
**a** hand extension,
**b** limp wrist,
**c** thumb abduction,
**d** paralysis

### Thumb Extension Test

Assesses a radial nerve lesion.

**Procedure:**   The patient is seated. The examiner grasps the patient's wrist with one hand and presses the thumb into adduction with the other hand. Then the patient is asked to extend or abduct both the metacarpophalangeal and interphalangeal joints of the thumb.

**Assessment:**   This test requires an intact radial nerve. Where this nerve is damaged, thumb extension will be weakened or will not be possible as a result of paralysis of the extensor pollicis longus and brevis. In patients with degenerative joint disease or rheumatoid arthritis in the joints of the thumb, this test generally produces pain in addition to demonstrating weakness. Simple nerve palsy without degenerative changes will not produce any joint symptoms.

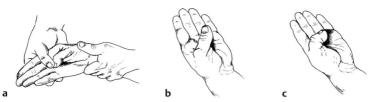

Fig. 4.**18a–c**   Thumb extension test:
**a** starting position,
**b** normal function,
**c** abnormal weakness in thumb extension

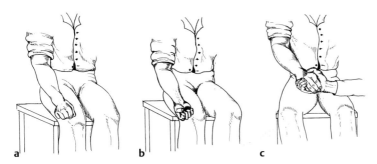

Fig. 4.**19a–c**   Supination test:
**a** starting position,
**b** normal supination,
**c** supination against resistance

### Supination Test

Assesses supinator pathology.

**Procedure:**   The patient is seated, holding the elbow slightly flexed and the forearm pronated. The elbow is held alongside the trunk to minimize motion in the shoulder. The patient is then asked to supinate his or her forearm, at first normally and then against the examiner's resistance.

**Assessment:**   Weakness or loss of supination of the forearm is a sign of supinator paralysis. The muscle is supplied by the deep branch of the radial nerve.

Care should be taken not to flex the elbow too much during this test. This is because the biceps also participates in supination with increasing flexion in the elbow. Despite the fact that both muscles are naturally

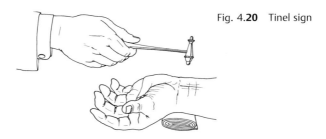

Fig. 4.**20**    Tinel sign

involved in supination, this would lead to false negative test results. This is because the biceps is involved in supination in increasing flexion, whereas the supinator has far greater influence on supination in extension.

### Tinel Sign

Indicates a median nerve lesion.

**Procedure:**  The patient's hand is slightly dorsiflexed; the dorsum of the wrist rests on a cushion on the examining table. The examiner taps the median nerve at the level of the wrist crease with a reflex hammer or the index finger.

**Assessment:**  Paresthesia and pain radiating into the hand and occasionally into the forearm as well are signs of a compression neuropathy of the median nerve (carpal tunnel syndrome). The tingling and paresthesia must be felt distal to the point of the pressure for a positive test. The test is also an indication of the rate of regeneration of the sensory fibers of the median nerve. The test will produce a false negative result in a chronic compression neuropathy in which nerve conductivity has already been severely reduced.

### Median Nerve Palsy Screening Test

Screening method for the assessment of median nerve palsy.

**Procedure:**  The patient is asked to oppose the tip of the thumb and the tip of the little finger. In the next step, the patient is asked to make a fist. Finally, the patient palmar flexes the hand slightly with the fingers extended.

**Assessment:**  Paralysis of the opponens pollicis makes it impossible to bring the tip of the thumb and the tip of the little finger into opposition.

Because of weakness of thumb opposition and flexion in the first three digits, the patient will be unable to make a fist. This produces a

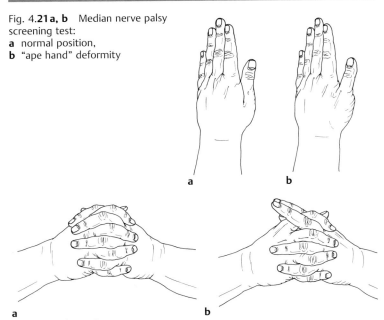

Fig. 4.**21 a, b**   Median nerve palsy screening test:
**a** normal position,
**b** "ape hand" deformity

Fig. 4.**22 a, b**   Ochsner test:
**a** normal position,
**b** the index and middle fingers extended due to weakness in the flexors

typical deformity in which only the ring and little fingers are flexed while the other digits remain extended.

Paralysis of the opponens, abductor pollicis brevis, and flexor pollicis brevis coupled with the antagonistic pull of the adductor pollicis cause the thumb to lie in the plane of the fingers. The thumbnail lies in the same plane as the fingernails, creating a deformity resembling an ape's hand, and the patient is unable to oppose the thumb.

### Ochsner Test

Indicates median nerve palsy.

**Procedure:**   The patient is asked to fold his or her hands with the fingers interlocked.

**Assessment:**   If median nerve palsy is present, the patient will be unable to flex the index and middle fingers due to partial paralysis of the flexor digitorum profundus.

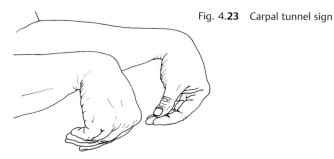

Fig. 4.**23**   Carpal tunnel sign

Fig. 4.**24**   Phalen test

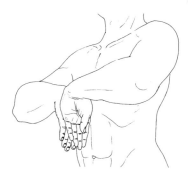

### Carpal Tunnel Sign

Indicates damage to the median nerve.

**Procedure:**  The patient is asked to keep his or her wrists completely flexed for 1–2 minutes.

**Assessment:**  Paresthesia that occurs or worsens in the region supplied by the median nerve is a sign of carpal tunnel syndrome.

### Phalen Test

Indicates damage to the median nerve.

**Procedure:**  The "wrist flexion sign" is evaluated by having the patient drop his or her hands into palmar flexion and then maintain this position for about 1–2 minutes. Pressing the dorsa of the hands together increases pressure in the carpal tunnel.

Fig. 4.**25a, b** Nail sign:
**a** normal,
**b** abnormal position due to weakened
opposition of the thumb

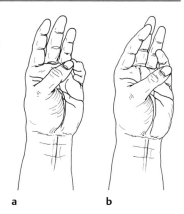

a                    b

**Assessment:** Pressing the dorsa of the hands together will often lead to paresthesia in the area supplied by the median nerve in normal patients as well, not just in those with carpal tunnel syndrome. Patients with carpal tunnel syndrome will experience worsening of symptoms in the Phalen test. Like the Tinel sign, this test can produce false negative results in the presence of chronic neuropathy.

### Nail Sign

Indicates damage to the median nerve.

**Procedure:** The patient is asked to touch his or her thumb to the tip of the little finger.

**Assessment:** Median nerve palsy will produce paralysis of the opponens pollicis. The thumb cannot be opposed but will only move along an arc in adduction toward the palm.

### Bottle Test

Indicates median nerve palsy.

**Procedure:** The patient is asked to grasp a bottle in each hand between the thumb and index finger.

**Assessment:** In paralysis of the abductor pollicis brevis, the web between the thumb and index finger will not be in contact with the surface of the bottle. The patient will be unable to hold the bottle between the thumb and index finger in such a way that the hand is in continuous contact with the circumference of the bottle.

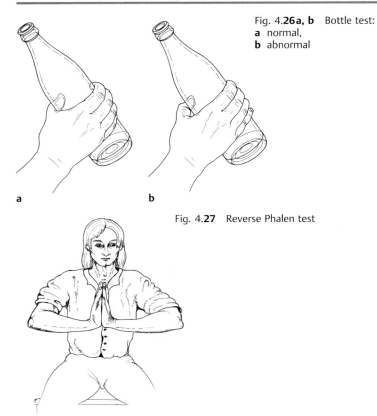

Fig. 4.**26a, b**    Bottle test:
**a**  normal,
**b**  abnormal

**a**

**b**

Fig. 4.**27**    Reverse Phalen test

### *Reverse Phalen Test*

Indicates carpal tunnel syndrome.

**Procedure:**   The seated patient is asked to press both hands together in maximum dorsiflexion and to maintain this position for one minute.

**Assessment:**   This position increases the pressure in the carpal tunnel. Paresthesia in the region supplied by the median nerve is a sign of carpal tunnel syndrome. The reverse Phalen test is less reliable than the Phalen test.

Fig. 4.**28a, b**
Pronation test:
**a** starting position,
**b** weakness in
   pronation of the
   right arm

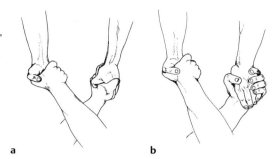

a                                b

### Pronation Test

Assessment of pronator teres and pronator quadratus pathology.

**Procedure:**   The patient is seated with both hands and forearms in supination on the examining table. The examiner asks the patient to pronate his or her forearms, initially normally and then against the resistance of the examiner's hand.

**Assessment:**   Weakness in active pronation against resistance in one arm as compared with the contralateral side indicates a median nerve lesion. The lesion normally lies at the level of the elbow. In the presence of a median nerve lesion distal to the elbow, the patient may be able to actively pronate the forearm against resistance because the pronator teres is still largely functional.

### Froment Sign

Indicates a cubital tunnel syndrome.

**Procedure:**   The patient is asked to hold a piece of paper between the thumb and index finger (pinch mechanism) against the pull of either the patient's contralateral hand or that of the examiner's hand. The muscle for this motion is the adductor pollicis, which is supplied by the ulnar nerve.

**Assessment:**   Where there is weakness or loss of function in this muscle, the interphalangeal joint of the thumb will be flexed due to contraction of the flexor pollicis brevis supplied by the median nerve. Occasional volar hypesthesia on the ring and little fingers is also a characteristic sign.

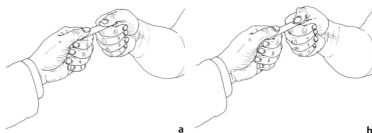

Fig. 4.**29a, b**  Froment sign:
**a** normal,
**b** abnormal

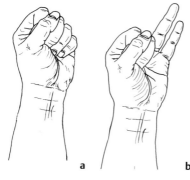

Fig. 4.**30a, b**  Ulnar nerve palsy screening test:
**a** normal,
**b** abnormal with loss of flexion in the ring and little fingers

### Ulnar Nerve Palsy Screening Test

Indicates ulnar nerve palsy.

**Procedure:**  The patient is asked to make a fist.

**Assessment:**  Where the ring and little fingers remain extended, flexion in the metacarpophalangeal and proximal interphalangeal joints of these finger is not possible. This is a sign of paralysis of the interossei. Patients with a long history of chronic ulnar nerve palsy will exhibit significant muscle atrophy between the fourth and fifth and first and second digital rays of the hand.

Fig. 4.**31** Intrinsic test

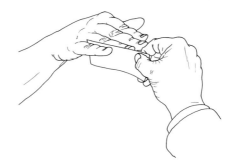

### Intrinsic Test

Indicates compression neuropathy of the ulnar nerve.

**Procedure:** The patient is asked to hold a piece of paper between the ring and little fingers. The examiner attempts to pull the piece of paper away from the patient.

**Assessment:** In the presence of ulnar nerve neuropathy, adduction in the little finger will be limited and the patient will be unable to hold on to the paper. The test should be performed on both hands for comparison. Compression neuropathy of the ulnar nerve can occur in the carpal tunnel, in the elbow, and in Guyon's canal in the wrist. A positive Tinel sign and paresthesia on the ring and little fingers are additional signs of compression. Complete ulnar nerve palsy results in loss of function in the intrinsic muscles of the hand. The fingers are then hyperextended in the metacarpophalangeal joints and flexed in the proximal and distal interphalangeal joints.

### O Test

**Procedure:** The pinch mechanism is a combined motion involving several muscles. Normally the thumb and index finger form the shape of an "O." With normal function in the muscles involved, the examiner will be unable to change the shape of the "O" by pulling on his or her own index finger inserted between the patient's thumb and index finger.

**Assessment:** In an anterior interosseous nerve syndrome with paralysis of the flexor digitorum profundus of the index finger and flexor pollicis longus, the thumb and index finger remain extended in the distal interphalangeal joints. The patient is then unable to form a proper "O" with the thumb and index finger.

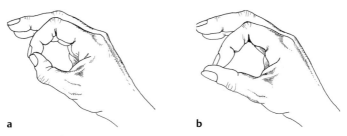

Fig. 4.**32a, b**   O test:
**a** normal,
**b** abnormal result with paralysis of the flexor digitorum profundus of the index
   finger and flexor pollicis longus

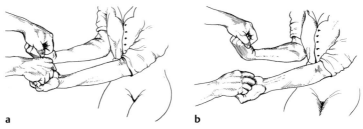

Fig. 4.**33a, b**   Wrist flexion test:
**a** normal,
**b** abnormal with weakness in active flexion of the left forearm

### *Wrist Flexion Test*

Assessment of distal nerve lesion in the forearm.

**Procedure:**   The patient is seated with both forearms supinated. The
examiner asks the patient to flex his or her wrists, first normally and
then against the resistance of the examiner's hands.

**Assessment:**   Weakness in active flexion against resistance indicates
paresis or paralysis of the flexors in the forearm, especially the flexor
carpi radialis. Weakness in this motion without resistance is a sign of
complete paralysis. Weakness in active flexion against resistance indicates a problem with the median nerve at the level of the elbow or
further proximally. Complete inability to flex the wrist against resistance could indicate a lesion involving both the median and ulnar
nerves.

# 5 Hip

Hip pain can have any number of causes. In children and adolescents, it is usually a sign of a serious disorder and therefore always requires a thorough diagnostic workup.

Patients usually report hip pain in the groin or posterior to the greater trochanter, occasionally radiating into the medial aspect of the thigh as far as the knee. For this reason, especially in children, a hip disorder can be easily misinterpreted as a knee disorder. The differential diagnosis should include disorders of the adductor tendons, lumbar spine, and, especially, the sacroiliac joints.

Many of the hip disorders associated with pain correlate with a certain age group. Frequent causes of pain in the hip include chronic hip dislocations and Legg–Calvé–Perthes disease in children and slipped capital femoral epiphysis in adolescents. In contrast, osteoarthritis of the hip is the primary cause of hip pain in adults.

Untreated or insufficiently treated congenital hip dislocation with persisting acetabular dysplasia is one of the most frequent causes of subsequent degenerative joint disease. Pain on walking, which patients usually describe as groin pain, is often attributable to hip dysplasia.

Aseptic necrosis of the femoral head, injuries, the "normal" aging process, and rheumatic and metabolic disorders are other disorders that can lead to degenerative hip disease. The hip joint is surrounded by a strong muscular envelope. Inspection alone will provide only a modest amount of diagnostic information about the condition of the joint. Even a significant joint effusion may escape detection. The position of the legs (flexion contracture of the hip, malrotation, or leg shortening) and the position of the spine (scoliosis or lordosis) are important in evaluating the pelvis; their abnormal positions may actually be caused by a hip disorder and can allow one to draw conclusions about the condition of the hip.

The normal pelvis is tilted anteriorly, producing lordosis in the lumbar spine. Contracture of the hip results in an abnormal position of the legs, pelvis, and back. This is usually more apparent when the patient is standing upright than when lying down. Increased lumbar lordosis can be due to a flexion contracture in the hip; this contracture may be compensated for by an increased anterior tilt of the pelvis and increased lordosis. Actual and apparent leg shortening also significantly influences leg position and gait. When examining leg length, one must

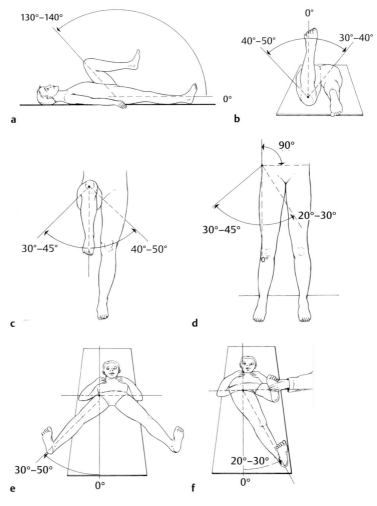

Fig. 5.**1a–f**
**a**    Flexion and extension of the hip, supine.
**b, c**  Internal and external rotation of the hip:
**b**    prone, with the hip extended,
**c**    supine, with the hip flexed.
**d**    Abduction and adduction of the hip.
**e, f**  Abduction and adduction of the hip.

consider the possibility of apparent lengthening or shortening due to an abduction or adduction contracture.

In the presence of an abduction contracture of the leg at the hip, the patient can only bring his or her legs into parallel alignment by tilting the pelvis. This pushes the normal hip upward, making that leg appear shortened. The adduction contracture has an analogous effect, although in this case the affected leg appears shortened. If the patient does not want to stand with one leg on tiptoe to compensate for the shortening, he or she will have to flex the contralateral knee. This produces an additional flexion in the hip that the patient can compensate for by increasing the anterior tilt of the pelvis.

Abnormal positioning of the pelvis due to hip disorders usually results in changes to the spine in the form of lumbar scoliosis and spinal torsion or a compensatory curvature of the posterior lumbar section of the spine.

Assessment of the patient's gait allows the examiner to identify gait abnormalities due to articular causes (osteoarthritis or inflammation) and/or muscular causes. In Duchenne antalgic gait, the patient attempts to reduce the load on the hip that causes the pain. In a Trendelenburg gait, weakness of the hip abductors, primarily the gluteal musculature, causes the pelvis to dip toward the unaffected side in the stance phase. In a compensatory limp with leg shortening, the upper body is shifted slightly over the leg in the stance phase. Otherwise, the gait is relatively smooth. Arthrodesis of the hip does not produce a true limp in the sense that the pelvis dips in the stance phase. Rather the increased tilt of the pelvis in the sagittal plane, as it moves from hyperlordosis into lumbar kyphosis, produces femoral anteversion in the swing phase.

Other function tests are of help in the closer assessment of hip disorders and in clarifying their cause and confirming the diagnosis.

## ■ Function Tests

### Muscle Traction Test

A compact quadriceps that cannot be stretched and shortened hamstrings increase retropatellar pressure. Shortening of the iliotibial tract can cause chronic pain on the lateral aspect and can also lead to patellofemoral joint dysfunction via its connection to the lateral retinaculum.

## Hip tests—Assessment

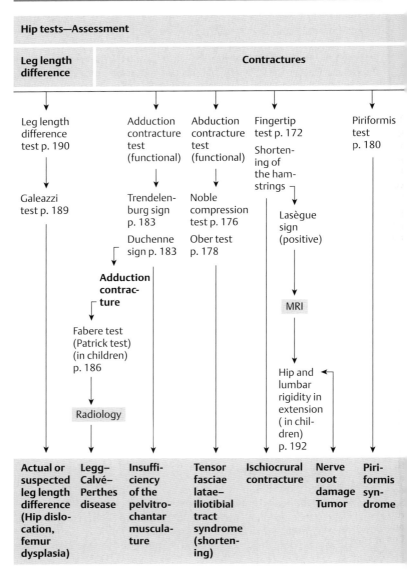

Fig. 5.**2**   Hip tests

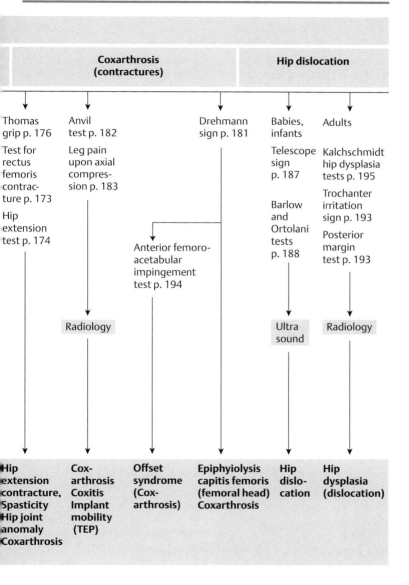

|  | Coxarthrosis (contractures) | | | Hip dislocation | |

Thomas
grip p. 176

Anvil
test p. 182

Drehmann
sign p. 181

Babies,
infants

Adults

Test for
rectus
femoris
contrac-
ture p. 173

Leg pain
upon axial
compres-
sion p. 183

Telescope
sign
p. 187

Kalchschmidt
hip dysplasia
tests p. 195

Hip
extension
test p. 174

Barlow
and
Ortolani
tests
p. 188

Trochanter
irritation
sign p. 193

Posterior
margin
test p. 193

Anterior femoro-
acetabular
impingement
test p. 194

Radiology

Ultra
sound

Radiology

Hip
extension
contracture,
Spasticity
Hip joint
anomaly
Coxarthrosis

Cox-
arthrosis
Coxitis
Implant
mobility
(TEP)

Offset
syndrome
(Cox-
arthrosis)

Epiphyiolysis
capitis femoris
(femoral head)
Coxarthrosis

Hip
dislo-
cation

Hip
dysplasia
(dislocation)

## Fingertip Test

Assesses contracture of the hamstrings.

**Procedure:**  The patient is seated, holding one leg (flexed at the hip and knee) close to the trunk with the ipsilateral arm. The other leg remains extended. The patient is requested to touch the toes of the extended leg with the fingertips of the free arm. This test is then repeated on the contralateral side.

**Assessment:**  In the presence of a hamstring contracture, the patient can only bring the fingertips into the general area of the foot and complains of "pulling" pain in the posterior thigh.

The test is positive where there is a difference between both sides and symptoms are present. Uniform, painless developmental shortening of the hamstrings is common. Restricted motion can result secondary to a spinal disorder or osteoarthritis of the hip.

**Note:**  Symptoms of nerve root irritation can be excluded by other tests. Shortened hamstrings increase retropatellar pressure and can therefore cause retropatellar symptoms.

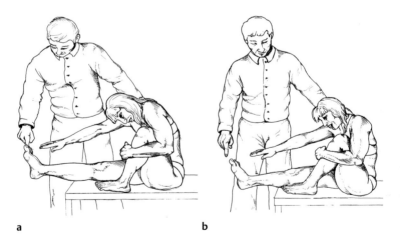

a                          b

Fig. 5.**3a, b**    Fingertip test:
**a** normal,
**b** abnormal with contracture of the hamstrings

## Test for Rectus Femoris Contracture

**Procedure:**   The patient is supine with the lower legs hanging over the edge of the examining table. The patient is requested to grasp one knee and pull it up against his or her chest. The examiner notes the angle that the hanging leg assumes. The test is repeated on the contralateral side.

**Assessment:**   In a contracture of the rectus femoris, drawing one knee closer to the chest will produce flexion in the other leg lying on the table; when this starts to happen will depend on the contracture. The test will also be positive in the presence of a flexion contracture of the hip due to a hip disorder, psoas irritation (psoas abscess), lumbar spine disorder, and change in pelvic inclination.

**Note:**   A contracture of the quadriceps increases the retropatellar pressure and may thus be the cause of retropatellar symptoms.

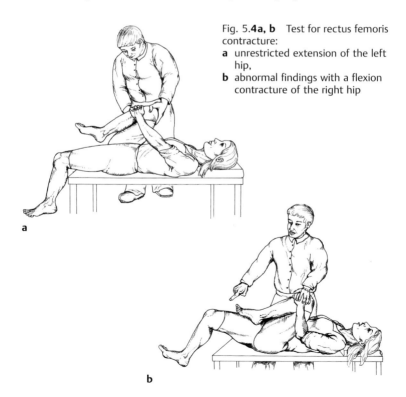

Fig. 5.**4a, b**   Test for rectus femoris contracture:
- **a** unrestricted extension of the left hip,
- **b** abnormal findings with a flexion contracture of the right hip

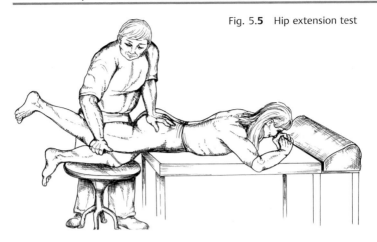

Fig. 5.**5**   Hip extension test

## Hip Extension Test

Assesses flexion contracture of the hip.

**Procedure:**   The patient is prone with both hips flexed over the edge of the examining table. The leg that is not being examined is held between the examiner's legs, supported on a chair, or simply allowed to hang down.

With one hand, the examiner immobilizes the patient's pelvis. With the other hand, he or she slowly extends the leg to be examined. The prone position fully compensates for the lumbar lordosis.

**Assessment:**   The point at which motion in the pelvis begins or the lumbar spine goes into lordosis indicates the endpoint of hip extension. The angle between the axis of the thigh and horizontal (the examining table) approximately indicates the flexion contracture in the hip. This test allows good assessment of a flexion contracture, especially in bilateral contractures (such as in spasticity).

## Iliotibial Tract Test

**Procedure:**   The patient lies in the lateral position. The leg to be examined is slightly adducted and the hip is slightly hyperextended.

The examiner places one hand on the distal iliotibial tract, which allows evaluation of muscle tone. With the forearm, the examiner grasps the lower leg near the ankle. Tension is placed on the iliotibial

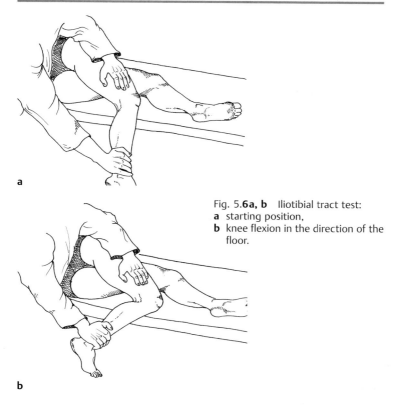

Fig. 5.**6a, b** Iliotibial tract test:
**a** starting position,
**b** knee flexion in the direction of the
floor.

tract by pressing the patient's lower leg toward the floor. The knee is then examined in various degrees of flexion.

**Assessment:** Increased tone as the knee approaches extension is readily detectable. However, flexing the knee reduces tension in the iliotibial tract as this moves the origin and insertion closer together. Careful palpation may detect fluctuations of the iliotibial tract near its insertion such as can occur in iliotibial tract friction syndrome or bursitis.

In severe shortening of the iliotibial tract or tensor fasciae latae, pain will also be felt at 30°–60° of flexion.

**Note:** Stretching the iliotibial tract often helps in lateral displacement of the patella with excessive lateral pressure.

## Thomas Grip

Assesses extension in the hip.

**Procedure:**   The patient is supine. The unaffected, contralateral leg is flexed at the hip until the lumbar lordosis disappears. This is verified by inserting one hand between the patient's lumbar spine and the examining table. With the patient in this position, the examiner immobilizes the pelvis in its normal position. The pelvis should exhibit about 12° of anterior inclination. This is what creates the lumbar lordosis. An increased flexion contracture in the hip can be compensated for by an increase in lumbar lordosis, in which case the patient only appears to assume a normal position.

**Assessment:**   Extension is only possible up to the neutral position (0°); the thigh lies flat on the surface of the examining table. Further flexion can tilt the pelvis further upright. So long as the leg being examined remains in contact with the examining table, the angle of pelvic tilt achieved corresponds to the maximum hyperextension of the hip.

In a flexion contracture, the hip being examined does not continue to lie extended on the examining table. Instead it moves along with the increasing hip flexion or pelvic tilt, taking on a position of increasing flexion. The flexion contracture can be quantified by measuring the angle that the flexed, affected leg forms with the examining table.

Contractures of the hip occur in osteoarthritis, inflammation, and articular deformities of the hips. They can also cause spinal disorders.

## Noble Compression Test

Evaluation of a contracture of the tensor fasciae latae.

**Procedure:**   The patient is supine. The examiner passively flexes the patient's knee 90° and the hip approximately 50°. With the fingers of the left hand, the examiner gently presses on the lateral femoral condyle. Maintaining the flexion in the hip and pressure on the lateral femoral condyle, the examiner then increasingly extends the knee passively. Once the knee is in about 40° of flexion, the patient is requested to fully extend the knee.

**Assessment:**   The tensor fasciae latae arises from the anterolateral margin of the ilium (anterior superior iliac spine). It is an anterior branch of the gluteus medius. Its tendon inserts into the anterior margin of the iliotibial tract, which reinforces the fascia lata of the thigh.

The tensor fasciae latae inserts into the iliotibial tract, which in turn inserts into the tubercle of Gerdy on the proximal tibia. Extending the

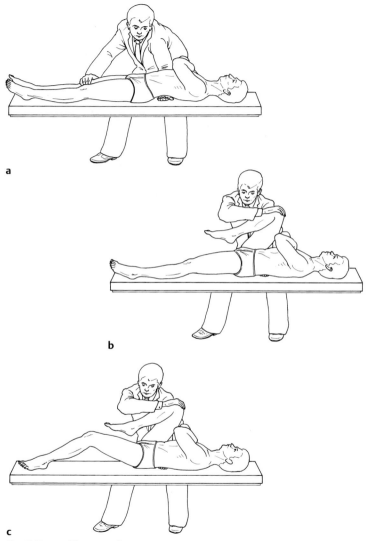

Fig. 5.**7a–c**  Thomas grip:
**a** starting position,
**b** normal,
**c** flexion contracture of the left hip

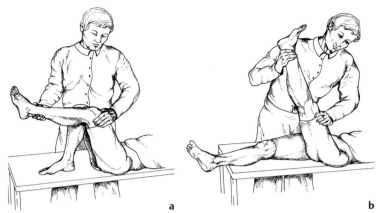

Fig. 5.**8a, b**   Noble compression test:
**a** starting position,
**b** extension

knee from 30° of flexion places maximum stress on the iliotibial tract.

Pain along the proximal and distal iliotibial tract suggests a contracture of the muscle or of the iliotibial tract itself. Pain in the posterior thigh that occurs with increasing extension is most likely indicative of a contracture of the hamstrings and should not be confused with a contracture of the tensor fasciae latae.

### Ober Test

Assesses a contracture of the iliotibial tract.

**Procedure:**   The patient lies on his or her unaffected side with the legs flexed at the hips and knees (to neutralize the lumbar lordosis). With one hand, the examiner grasps the patient's affected leg while stabilizing the pelvis with the other hand. The examiner then passively extends the hip, which brings the femur into line with the pelvis and thus immobilizes the iliotibial tract at the level of the greater trochanter. The leg is then adducted from this position.

**Assessment:**   If the iliotibial tract is shortened, the degree of hip adduction it allows will be limited in direct proportion to the degree of shortening. The test can also be performed in such a manner that the examiner abducts the extended leg and then lets go of it from a certain degree of abduction. If the leg fails to drop back into an appropriate

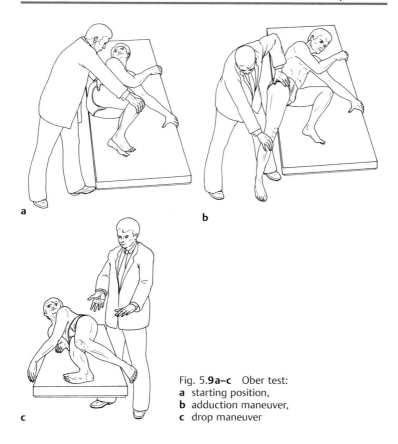

Fig. 5.**9a–c** Ober test:
**a** starting position,
**b** adduction maneuver,
**c** drop maneuver

adduction position or if flexion or rotation suddenly occurs, then a contracture of the iliotibial tract is present. Ober originally described the test with the knee flexed. However, the iliotibial band has a greater traction placed on it when the knee is extended. Also, when the knee is flexed during the test greater stress is placed on the femoral nerve. If neurologic signs (i.e., pain and paresthesia) occur during the test, the examiner should consider pathology affecting the femoral nerve. Likewise tenderness over the greater trochanter should lead the examiner to consider trochanterica bursitis.

When the knee is flexed to 90° accompanied by hip flexion the examiner then applies pressure with the thumb to the lateral femoral epicondyle. While the pressure is maintained the patient slowly extends the knee. At approximately 30° of flexion if the patient complains of severe pain over the lateral femur condyle a positive test is indicated. The patient usually says it is the same pain that accompanies the patient's activity (e.g., running). This test is also called the Noble compression test or iliotibial band friction test. It can be also performed with the patient supine in cases of chronic inflammation of the iliotibial band near its insertion.

**Note:** A shortened iliotibial tract leads to chronic pain in the lateral thigh and to functional impairment in the patellofemoral joint through its attachment with the lateral patellar retinaculum.

### Piriformis Test

**Procedure:** The patient lies in the lateral position with the test leg uppermost. The patient flexes the hip of that leg to 60° with the knee flexed. The examiner stabilizes the hip with one hand and applies downward pressure to the knee.

**Assessment:** If the piriformis is tight, pain is elicited in the muscle. If the piriformis is pinching the sciatic nerve, pain results in the buttock and sciatica may be experienced by the patient. Resisted lateral rotation with the muscle under traction (hip medially rotated) can cause the same sciatica. In about 15% of the population the sciatic nerve, all or in part, passes through the piriformis rather than below it. These people are more likely to suffer from this relatively rare piriformis syndrome.

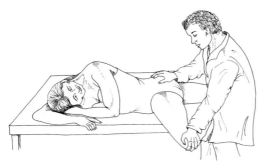

Fig. 5.**10** Piriformis test: the patient lies in the lateral position with the leg uppermost. The hip and knee are flexed

## Drehmann Sign

Indicates a hip disorder.

**Procedure:** The patient is supine. The examiner grasps the patient's foot and knee and flexes the knee.

A hip disorder is present when flexion produces increasing external rotation in the hip. The motion may be painless or it may cause pain.

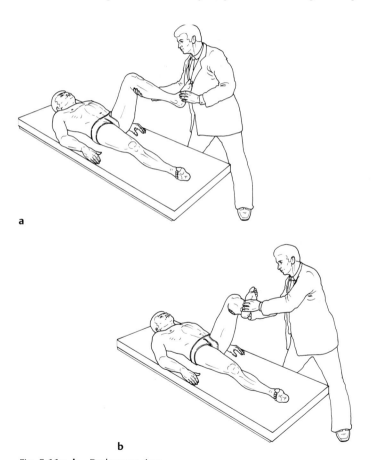

Fig. 5.**11a, b** Drehmann sign:
**a** knee and hip flexion,
**b** external rotation of the hip

**Assessment:**  In adolescents, a positive Drehmann sign occurs primarily in the presence of a slipped capital femoral epiphysis. This causes the thigh to move into increasing compensatory external rotation as the hip is flexed.

However, a hip infection, incipient osteoarthritis, or a tumor may also produce positive test results.

### Anvil Test

Indicates hip disease.

**Procedure:**  The patient is supine with legs extended. The examiner raises the extended leg slightly with one hand and hits the heel axially with the fist of the other hand.

**Assessment:**  The force of the blow is transmitted to the hip. Pain in the groin or in the thigh adjacent to the hip suggests hip disease (such as osteoarthritis of the hip or inflammation), or a femoral fracture. In total hip arthroplasty patients, it suggests implant loosening (groin pain suggests loosening of the acetabular component, whereas pain in the lateral thigh suggests loosening of the femoral stem).

Symptoms in the lumbar spine occur in intervertebral disk disease or in rheumatoid spine disorders.

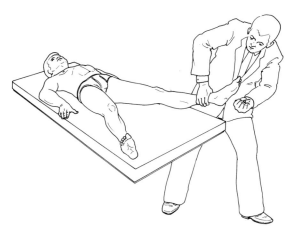

Fig. 5.**12**
Anvil test

## Leg Pain upon Axial Compression

Variation of the anvil test; indicates hip disease.

**Procedure:**   The patient is supine with one leg extended and the other flexed at the knee. The lateral malleolus of the flexed leg lies just superior to the patella of the contralateral leg. The examiner grasps the distal thigh of the flexed leg with both hands and compresses it axially.

**Assessment:**   This motion compresses the hip joint and the affected side of the pelvis.

Pain in the groin suggests hip disease such as osteoarthritis of the hip. In total hip arthroplasty patients, it suggests implant loosening.

Symptoms in the lumbar spine occur in intervertebral disk disease or in rheumatoid spine disorders.

## Trendelenburg Sign/Duchenne Sign

Tests pelvic and trochanteric muscle function.

**Procedure:**   The examiner stands behind the standing patient. The patient is requested to raise one leg by flexing the knee and hip.

**Assessment:**   In the single leg stance, the pelvic and trochanteric musculature (gluteus medius and gluteus minimus) on the weight-bearing side contract and elevate the pelvis on the unsupported side, holding it nearly horizontal.

Fig. 5.**13**   Leg pain upon axial compression

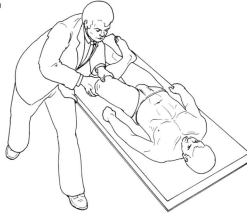

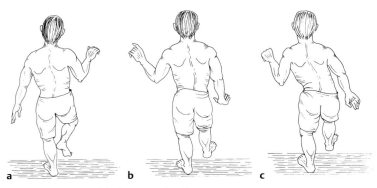

Fig. 5.**14a–c**   Trendelenburg sign/Duchenne sign:
**a** normal hip: patient can lift the pelvis by contracting the pelvic and trochanteric musculature on the weight-bearing side;
**b** insufficiency of the pelvic and trochanteric musculature causes the pelvic to dip toward the normal nonweight-bearing side (positive Trendelenburg sign),
**c** insufficiency of the pelvic and trochanteric musculature can be partially compensated for by shifting the body's center of gravity toward the weight-bearing leg (Duchenne sign)

Table 5.**1**   Grading of the Trendelenburg sign (from Hoppenfeld 1982)

| | |
|---|---|
| Negative | Patient can lift the pelvis on the nonweight-bearing side |
| Weakly positive | Patient can maintain the position of the pelvis on the nonweight-bearing side but not lift it |
| Positive | Pelvis on the nonweight-bearing side drops visibly |

This process allows uniform gait. Where the gluteal muscles are compromised (weakened as a result of a hip dislocation, due to paralysis, or following multiple hip operations) with functional deficits, they are no longer able to support the pelvis on the weight-bearing side. The pelvis then drops down on the normal, non-weight-bearing side (positive Trendelenburg sign). The patient will exhibit a typical duck-like waddling gait, especially in a bilateral condition (as in bilateral hip dislocation).

The drop in the pelvis toward the unaffected side also shifts the body's center of gravity in that direction. Patients usually compensate by shifting the body toward the weight-bearing leg (Duchenne sign). Reasons for insufficiency of the pelvic and trochanteric musculature:

- Genuine weakness (paresis or paralysis)
- Reduced distance between origin and insertion (hip dislocation, high-riding greater trochanter, varus osteotomy, Legg–Calvé–Perthes disease)
- Altered mechanics (shortened femoral neck, increased anteversion)
- Pain

## Anteversion Test

**Procedure:** The patient lies prone with the knee flexed 90°. The examiner palpates the greater trochanter of the femur. The hip is then passively rotated medially and laterally until the greater trochanter is parallel with the examining table or reaches its most lateral position.

**Assessment:** The degree of an anteversion can then be estimated based on the angle of the lower leg with the vertical. The precision of this measurement performed by an experienced examiner is comparable to radiographic measurement.

**Note:** Anteversion of the hip is measured by the angle made by the femoral neck with the femoral condyles.

It is the degree of forward projection of the femoral neck from the coronal plane of the shaft and it decreases during the growing period. At birth the mean angle is approximately 30°; in the adult the mean angle is 8°–15°. Increased anteversion leads to squinting patella and toeing in.

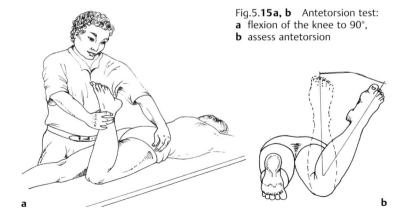

Fig.5.**15a, b** Antetorsion test:
**a** flexion of the knee to 90°,
**b** assess antetorsion

a            b

### Fabere Test (Patrick Test) for Legg–Calvé–Perthes Disease

**Procedure:**  The child is supine with one leg extended and the other flexed at the knee. The lateral malleolus of the flexed leg lies across the other leg superior to the patella. The test may also be performed so that the foot of the flexed leg is in contact with the medial aspect of the knee of the contralateral leg. The flexed leg is then pressed or allowed to fall further into abduction.

**Assessment:**  Normally the knee of the abducted leg will almost touch the examining table. The examiner makes comparative measurements of the distance between the knee and the table on both sides. On the side of the positive Patrick sign, motion is impaired, the adductors are tensed, and the patient feels pain when the leg is further abducted past

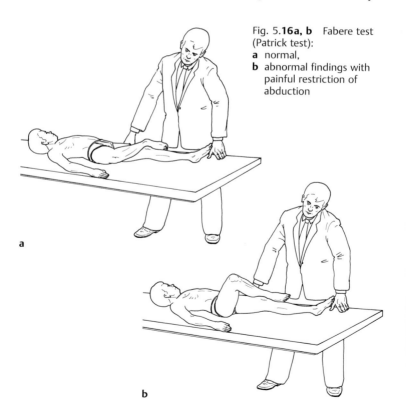

Fig. 5.**16a, b**   Fabere test (Patrick test):
**a** normal,
**b** abnormal findings with painful restriction of abduction

the starting position in limited abduction. Pain in the groin can be a sign of Legg–Calvé–Perthes disease.

Legg–Calvé–Perthes disease is regarded as belonging to the group of aseptic avascular necroses. The disease manifests itself in the epiphysis, metaphysis, and apophysis of the long bones and in the tarsal and carpal bones that ossify within the cartilage. Legg–Calvé–Perthes disease is the most common form of aseptic bone necrosis. It occurs primarily between the ages of 3 and 12 years, with peak occurrence between the ages of 4 and 8 years. In the early stages of the disease, children tire quickly and begin to limp slightly. They complain of slight pain in the hip; occasionally they only complain of knee pain.

### Telescope Sign

Indicates congenital hip dislocation.

**Procedure:**  The examiner grasps the affected leg with one hand and passively flexes the hip and knee. The other hand rests posterolateral to the hip. The examiner palpates the greater trochanter with the thumb of this hand and the motion of the femoral head with the index finger. The hand guiding the leg alternately applies axial compression and traction to the femur.

**Assessment:**  In a hip dislocation, the leg will appear to shorten or lengthen. The palpating hand follows the motion of the greater trochanter and femoral head into the dislocated position and back to reduction.

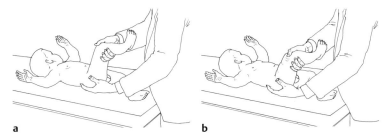

Fig. 5.**17a, b**   Telescope sign:
**a** leg "shortening" on axial compression,
**b** leg "lengthening" on axial traction

## Barlow and Ortolani Tests

Assess hip instability in infants.

**Procedure:**  With the infant supine, the examiner passively flexes one leg, immobilizing the pelvis. The other hand grasps the knee and thigh of the leg to be examined in such a manner that the index finger and thumb rest inferior to the inguinal fold.

With the thigh initially in extreme adduction, the examiner carefully exerts axial pressure while simultaneously pressing the thigh into abduction from the medial side. The fingers provide controlled resilient resistance to this motion. Instability in the hip will be palpable as the direction of force changes between the fingers and thumb. This is the Barlow dislocation test.

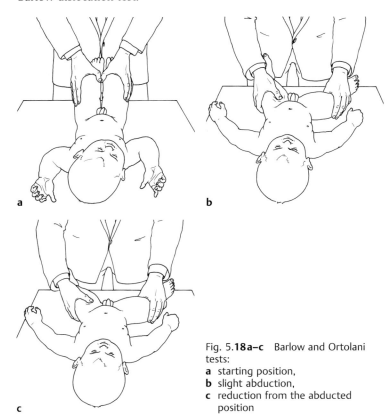

Fig. 5.**18a–c**   Barlow and Ortolani tests:
**a** starting position,
**b** slight abduction,
**c** reduction from the abducted position

In the second phase of the examination, the examiner slowly abducts the thigh while maintaining axial compression. If the femoral head was pushed out of the center of the acetabulum during the first phase (Barlow test), the examiner can now reduce it into the acetabulum with a palpable snap by pressing on the greater trochanter with the fingers. This is known as the Ortolani "click."

This test should be repeated separately for each leg.

**Assessment:**  The examination detects instability of the hip and also allows one to define the degree of instability present. Toennis differentiates four grades of instability:

Grade I:  Slightly unstable hip without a snap.

Grade II:  Dislocatable hip. The hip can be fully or largely reduced by abduction alone (with a snap).

Grade III:  Hip that can be dislocated and reduced.

Grade IV:  Dislocated hip that cannot be reduced. The acetabulum is empty, and the femoral head can be palpated posteriorly; abduction is severely limited and reduction is not possible.

**Note:**  A "dry click" without dislocation can often be provoked during in the first days of life, but disappears thereafter.

The Barlow and Ortolani test is particularly useful in newborns 2–3 weeks old. The Ludloff–Hohmann test is an alternative in slightly older children. With the hip flexed and abducted, spontaneous knee flexion will normally occur as a result of the physiologic tension in the hamstrings. A knee that can be fully extended with the hip flexed and abducted suggests an unstable hip.

## Galeazzi Test

Assesses leg length difference.

**Procedure:**  The patient is supine with the knees flexed 90° and the soles of the feet flat on the examining table. The examiner assesses the position of both knees from the end of the table and from the side.

**Assessment:**  Normally both knees are at the same level. Where one knee is higher than the other, either the tibia of that side is longer or the contralateral tibia is shorter. Where one knee projects farther forward than the other, either that femur is longer or the contralateral femur is shorter. The test for assessment of femur length is indicated as an additional test for evaluating hip dislocation. However, in such a case there is only an apparent difference in length; the femurs are the same length but one thigh appears shorter due to the hip dislocation.

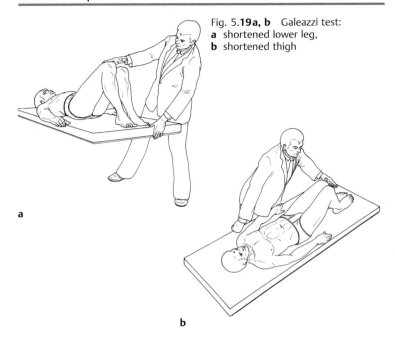

Fig. 5.**19a, b**   Galeazzi test:
**a** shortened lower leg,
**b** shortened thigh

a

b

Note that the Galeazzi test will yield a false-negative result in cases of bilateral hip dislocation.

### Leg Length Difference Test

Assesses actual and functional leg length differences.

**Procedure:**   Measurement of an actual difference in leg length is performed with the patient standing by placing shims of varying thickness (0.5, 1, 2 cm) underneath the shorter leg until the pelvic obliquity is fully compensated.

**Assessment:**   Compensation of the pelvic obliquity is usually readily apparent, especially when the patient bends forward from a standing position. With the pelvis horizontal, the leg length difference corresponds to the total height of the shims placed beneath the foot. Evaluating leg length difference by palpating the iliac crests from behind the patient is often imprecise. Often the iliac wings (iliac crests) will not be at the same level although radiographic findings confirm identical leg length and a normal vertical spine.

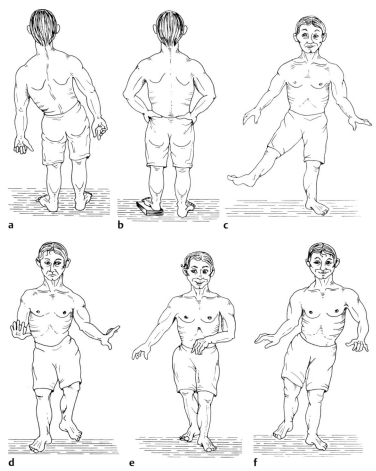

Fig. 5.**20a–f**   Leg length difference test.

**a, b**  Actual shortening of the leg: The legs appear equally long with the patient standing. Shortening of the left leg is compensated for by pelvic obliquity and scoliotic posture (**a**). The pelvic obliquity and scoliotic posture can be eliminated by placing shims under the leg (**b**).

**c, d**  Functional lengthening of the leg: Abduction contracture on the right side (**c**). The pelvis dips toward the affected side. The normal leg appears shortened and the affected leg lengthened (**d**).

**e, f**  Functional shortening of the leg: Adduction contracture on the right side (**e**). The affected leg appears shortened and the normal leg lengthened (**f**).

Asymmetric iliac wings are frequently encountered in conditions such as hip dysplasia. The iliac wing on the dysplastic side is usually smaller. Often only a pelvis radiograph obtained with the patient standing and showing the sacrum and lower lumbar spine will allow one to draw reliable conclusions about the type and severity of the leg length difference.

Where placement of shims cannot compensate the pelvic obliquity, the patient has a fixed deformity of one or more joints or a fixed scoliosis leading to a functional leg length difference. This functional difference occurs as a result of a flexion or adduction contracture in the hip. The pelvis dips toward the normal side; the normal leg appears lengthened and the affected leg shortened.

An abduction contracture in the hip causes a functional leg length difference. The pelvis dips toward the affected side; the normal leg appears shortened and the affected leg lengthened. An actual leg length difference is best evaluated and measured with the patient standing, a functional difference with the patient supine.

## Hip and Lumbar Rigidity in Extension

Indicates spinal cord disease and intervertebral disk pathology in children.

**Procedure:**   The child is supine. The examiner lifts the child's legs.

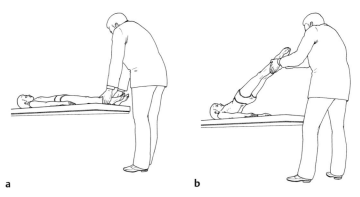

Fig. 5.**21a, b**   Hip and lumbar rigidity in extension:
**a** starting position,
**b** abnormal findings

**Assessment:** Reflexive rigidity that maintains hip extension when the child's legs are lifted is a sign of a spinal cord lesion such as a tumor, compression of the spinal cord as in spondylolisthesis, or nerve root compression as in intervertebral disk extrusion.

### Trochanter Irritation Sign

Test of abductor function, indicative of hip dysplasia.

**Procedure:** The patient lies on the normal side. In this lateral position, the patient performs bicycle pedaling motions in slight abduction.

**Assessment:** Pain felt over the greater trochanter and gluteal musculature is indicative of exercise pain in the abductors, which in turn can suggest hip dysplasia or bursitis trochanterica. This test is only performed in patients with a history of exercise pain in the abductors.

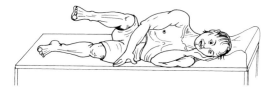

Fig. 5.**22** Trochanter irritation sign

### Posterior Margin Test

Indicates a lesion of the posterior acetabular labrum.

**Procedure:** With the patient supine, the hip is forcibly flexed, abducted, and externally rotated. Then it is extended in adduction and internal rotation.

**Assessment:** In this maneuver, motion of the femoral head places compressive and shear stresses on the capsule-labrum complex. Pain felt in the posterolateral region of the hip is a sign of a posterior capsular and/or labral lesion.

A diagnostic infiltration test (intraarticular injection of 10 ml of 1% xylocaine) can differentiate between intraarticular and extraarticular pain patterns. Where a labral lesion is present, painfully restricted motion should be limited to flexion and rotation and the capsular pattern, and the positive labrum provocation tests should be completely normal or greatly improved immediately after infiltration.

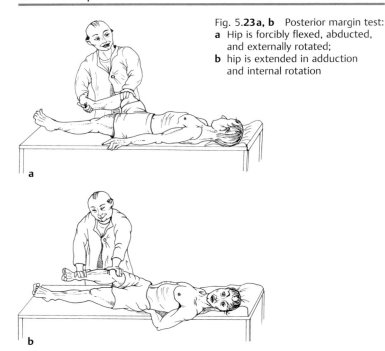

Fig. 5.**23a, b**   Posterior margin test:
**a** Hip is forcibly flexed, abducted, and externally rotated;
**b** hip is extended in adduction and internal rotation

## Anterior Femoroacetabular Impingement Test

The test demonstrates involvement of the acetabular rim and femoral head–neck junction.

**Procedure:**   The patient is supine. The examiner passively flexes, adducts, and internally rotates the patient's hip

**Assessment:**   Symptomatic femoroacetabular impingement is characterized by painfully limited internal rotation and flexion. Pain felt in the anteromedial and anterolateral region of the hip.

The impingement occurs when bony prominences of the femoral head–neck junction (Cam impingement) and/or the acetabular rim (Pincer impingement) lead to early contact, causing substantial labral and prearthrotic chondral damage, particularly in young and active adults.

A deep acetabulum, post-slip and Legg–Calvé–Perthes deformity, a retroversion of the acetabulum, and a decreased anteversion of the femur also caused restricted internal rotation and flexion of the hip.

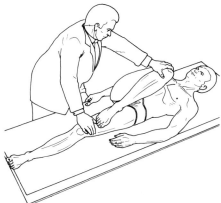

Fig. 5.**24**  Anterior femoroace-tabular impingement test

## Kalchschmidt Hip Dysplasia Tests

Assess symptoms caused by hip dysplasia.

Most patients with symptoms due to hip dysplasia report pain with weightbearing felt in the groin or the region of the greater trochanter. However, there are patients who cannot clearly identify the anatomic region of the symptoms and complain of pain in the lower back, buttock, and thigh.

The following tests are helpful where clinical and radiographic evidence suggests painful hip dysplasia:

### Test 1

With the patient standing on the painful leg and the examiner guiding the patient's shoulders, the examiner turns the patient's body so that the affected hip is in maximum external rotation. Backward bending also hyperextends the hip.

Where symptoms are attributable to hip dysplasia, this posture will cause groin pain. When the patient then bends forward and the hip is brought into internal rotation by the examiner's guiding of the patient's shoulders, the pain disappears.

### Test 2

The patient is prone (a sandbag may also be placed under the knee). While pressing on the patient's buttock, the examiner passively flexes the patient's knee 90° and applies increasing resilient pressure to externally rotate the thigh.

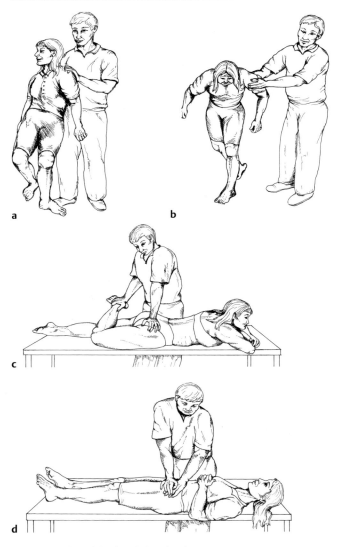

Fig. 5.**25a–d**   Kalchschmidt hip dysplasia tests:
**a, b**   Test 1,
**c**      Test 2,
**d**      Test 3

Where symptoms are attributable to hip dysplasia, the patient will report pain in the groin region. This test provides useful diagnostic information when both sides are compared, and it is easy to perform.

### Test 3

The patient is supine. First the examiner palpates the hip beneath the anterior inferior iliac spine. The examiner then places increasing pressure on the femoral head by pressing with the hypothenar eminence of the extended arm.

Where symptoms are attributable to hip dysplasia, the patient will report pain. This test provides useful diagnostic information, especially when both sides are compared. Often, the examiner will observe that performing the test presses an eccentric, anteriorly displaced femoral head back into the acetabulum.

# 6 Knee

Our knowledge of the knee has expanded significantly over the last few decades. New information about anatomy, biomechanics, and pathophysiology has improved the detection and treatment of knee disorders. Injuries to the knee, particularly in conjunction with sports activities, have become a major focus of interest.

Noninvasive modalities such as ultrasound, computed tomography, and magnetic resonance imaging today allow precise assessment of diseased and injured structures in the knee. Diagnostic arthroscopy has evolved into a surgical method of treatment.

Diagnostic assessment of knee symptoms begins with history taking and physical examination. Anteroposterior and lateral radiographs of the knee together with an axial view of the patella and trochlear groove are required to detect changes in bony structures right at the start.

It is very important to identify the location and type of pain as well its duration or when it occurs (pain with weightbearing, joint blockade, etc.). Inspection and evaluation of axial deviations (genu valgum, genu varum, genu recurvatum, or a flexion deformity), swelling of the knee, and muscle atrophy provide information about the possible causes of joint symptoms. Palpation then allows the examiner to identify diseased joint structures with greater accuracy and assess them in greater detail. Clinical tests of passive and active motion, some of which entail complex motions, also aid in making a diagnosis. Understanding how the accident occurred is important for diagnosing knee injuries. The type and severity of the injury are dependent on the direction, duration, and intensity of the trauma and on the position of the joint at the time of the injury.

Sports injuries and developmental anomalies (axial deviations, malformation of the patella, etc.) are the most common causes of knee complaints in children and young adults. For example, Osgood–Schlatter disease should be suspected when an adolescent engaged in a jumping sport in school athletics complains of pain in the tibial tuberosity. In older adolescents, one should suspect patellar tendinitis ("jumper's knee"). Degenerative damage to the meniscus can lead to sudden meniscus symptoms with impingement without an identifiable causative event even in early adulthood. In older patients, incipient or advanced wear in the joint due to aging processes, posttraumatic conditions, occupational stresses, and congenital or acquired deformities is most often responsible for knee symptoms. Diffuse knee pain occurring in an older patient in the absence of trauma is almost invariably a sign of meniscus degeneration or joint wear. Swelling and a sensation of heat in the knee are normally present as well. Patients with retropatellar arthritis complain of pain on climbing stairs and walking downhill, occasionally accompanied by a feeling of instability. Patients with Baker cysts report pain in the popliteal fossa.

Aside from these characteristic descriptions of pain, any uncharacteristic pain described by the patient should be carefully assessed. The differential diagnosis must include disorders of the adjacent joints. Patients with osteoarthritis of the hip will often report pain radiating into the knee. Changes in the sacroiliac joints or lumbar spine, leg shortening, axial deviations, and ankle deformities can also cause knee symptoms.

Disorders of other organ systems should also be considered when assessing distal neurovascular dysfunction. The knee is affected in 60% of all cases in rheumatoid arthritis. Lyme disease should also be considered as a possible cause of isolated arthritis of the knee. A thorough history and extensive laboratory diagnostic studies are helpful in the differential diagnosis of such knee disorders.

## ■ Range of Motion in the Knee (Neutral-Zero Method)

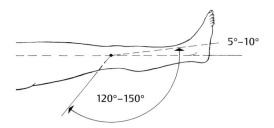

**Fig. 6.1** Flexion and extension. Internal and external rotation do not occur in extension. In 90° of knee flexion with the lower leg hanging freely, the knee exhibits a range of motion from 10° of internal rotation to up to 25° of external rotation

## Knee tests—Assessment

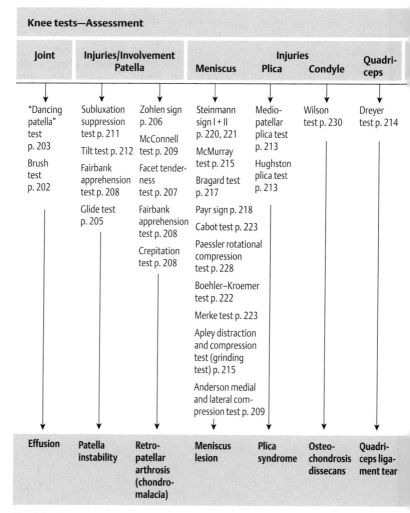

| Joint | Injuries/Involvement Patella | | Injuries | | | Quadri-ceps |
| | | | Meniscus | Plica | Condyle | |
|---|---|---|---|---|---|---|
| "Dancing patella" test p. 203<br><br>Brush test p. 202 | Subluxation suppression test p. 211<br><br>Tilt test p. 212<br><br>Fairbank apprehension test p. 208<br><br>Glide test p. 205 | Zohlen sign p. 206<br><br>McConnell test p. 209<br><br>Facet tenderness test p. 207<br><br>Fairbank apprehension test p. 208<br><br>Crepitation test p. 208 | Steinmann sign I + II p. 220, 221<br><br>McMurray test p. 215<br><br>Bragard test p. 217<br><br>Payr sign p. 218<br><br>Cabot test p. 223<br><br>Paessler rotational compression test p. 228<br><br>Boehler–Kroemer test p. 222<br><br>Merke test p. 223<br><br>Apley distraction and compression test (grinding test) p. 215<br><br>Anderson medial and lateral compression test p. 209 | Medio-patellar plica test p. 213<br><br>Hughston plica test p. 213 | Wilson test p. 230 | Dreyer test p. 214 |
| Effusion | Patella instability | Retro-patellar arthrosis (chondro-malacia) | Meniscus lesion | Plica syndrome | Osteo-chondrosis dissecans | Quadri-ceps liga-ment tear |

Fig. 6.2   Knee tests

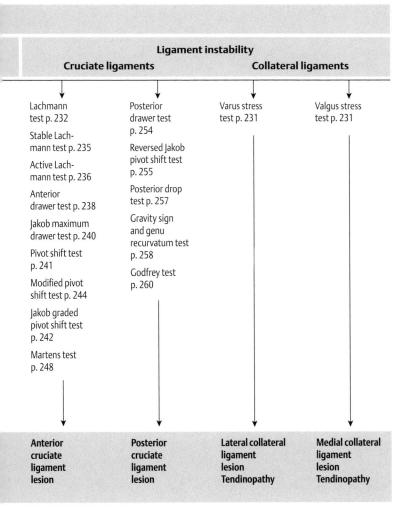

**Ligament instability**

**Cruciate ligaments**

Lachmann
test p. 232

Stable Lach-
mann test p. 235

Active Lach-
mann test p. 236

Anterior
drawer test p. 238

Jakob maximum
drawer test p. 240

Pivot shift test
p. 241

Modified pivot
shift test p. 244

Jakob graded
pivot shift test
p. 242

Martens test
p. 248

**Anterior
cruciate
ligament
lesion**

Posterior
drawer test
p. 254

Reversed Jakob
pivot shift test
p. 255

Posterior drop
test p. 257

Gravity sign
and genu
recurvatum test
p. 258

Godfrey test
p. 260

**Posterior
cruciate
ligament
lesion**

**Collateral ligaments**

Varus stress
test p. 231

**Lateral collateral
ligament
lesion
Tendinopathy**

Valgus stress
test p. 231

**Medial collateral
ligament
lesion
Tendinopathy**

# ■ Knee Swelling

When assessing swelling, the examiner must determine the type and amount of swelling that are present.

The examiner must differentiate between swelling and synovial thickening. Normally the knee contains 1–2 ml synovial fluid.

If the swelling consists of blood (hemarthrosis) it may be caused by a ligament tear, osteochondral fracture, or peripheral meniscus tear.

"Blood" swelling comes on very quickly (within 1–2 hours) and the shin becomes very taut. On palpation it has a "doughy" feeling and is relatively hard to the touch. The joint surface fells warm. Normally synovial fluid swelling caused by joint irritation occurs in 8–24 hours.

The feeling within the joint is a fluctuating or "boggy" feeling. The joint surface feels warm and tender. Swelling usually occurs with activity and disappears after a few days of inactivity.

### Brush (Stroke, Wipe) Test

For assessing minimal effusion.

**Procedure:**   The patient lies supine. The examiner places one hand and index finger on the lateral leg distal and medial to the patella. With the other hand the examiner presses the superior recess moving distally from a proximal and lateral position.

**Assessment:**   In slight joint effusion a wave of fluid and spreading of the forefingers and the thumb may be felt.

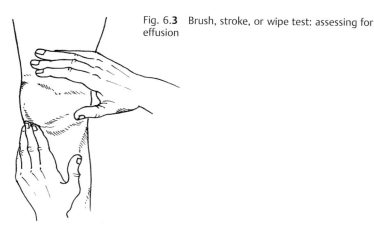

Fig. 6.**3**   Brush, stroke, or wipe test: assessing for effusion

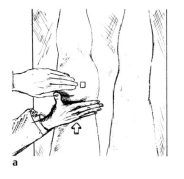

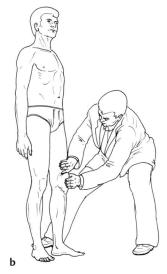

Fig. 6.**4a, b**   "Dancing patella" test:
**a** with the patient supine,
**b** with the patient standing

### "Dancing Patella" Test

Indicates effusion in the knee.

**Procedure:**   The patient is supine or standing. With one hand, the examiner smoothes the suprapatellar pouch from proximal to distal while pressing the patella against the femur with the other hand or moving it medially and laterally with slight pressure.

**Assessment:**   Resilient resistance (a dancing patella) is abnormal and suggests effusion in the knee.

## ■ Patella

### Patellar Chondropathy (Chondromalacia, Anterior Knee Pain)

Malformations of the patella (patellar dysplasia) and of the trochlear groove (flattening of the lateral femoral condyle) and abnormal position of the patella (patella alta or lateral displacement) create abnormal mechanical stresses in the trochlear groove and with time can lead to arthritis. Aging processes, injuries (such cartilage impingement or fractures), recurrent patellar dislocations, and inflammations (as in gout or rheumatism) are other factors that can lead to osteoarthritis.

Patients complain of retropatellar symptoms, pain in extreme knee flexion and when climbing stairs, and a feeling of instability.

Upon clinical examination, the patella will not be very mobile. The patient feels pain when the patella is pressed against the knee or moved, and the margins of the patella are painful. The apprehension test is usually positive.

Other factors promoting dislocation of the patella include axial deviation (genu valgum), malrotation of the tibia, and weak capsular ligaments. Patellar hypermobility in particular leads to impaired nutrient supply to the cartilage, accelerating cartilage damage. In patellar hypermobility with recurrent subluxation, the constant microtrauma causes cartilage lesions.

## Q-Angle Test

The Q-angle is defined as the angle between the quadriceps muscle (primarily the rectus femoris) and the patellar tendon.

It corresponds to the physiologic valgus angle of the femoral shaft.

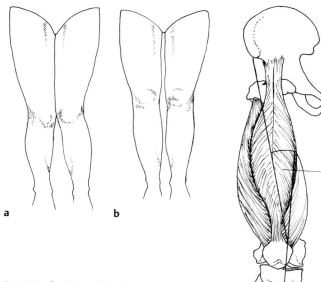

Fig. 6.**5a, b**   Q-angle test:
**a**  leg axis normal,
**b**  left: genu valgum with increased Q-angle,
**c**  defining the Q-angle

This creates a lateral pull on the patella. This tendency is a factor in habitual patellar dislocation and in patella syndrome. It also creates problems in total knee arthroplasty.

**Procedure:**  A line is drawn from the anterior superior iliac spine to the midpoint of the patella and from the tibial tubercle to the midpoint of the patella. The angle formed by the crossing of these two lines is called the Q-angle.

The hip and the foot should be placed in a neutral position, because different hip and foot positions alter the Q-angle.

**Assessment:**  Normally the Q-angle is 13° for males and 18° for females when the knee is straight. Any angle less than 13° may be associated with patellofemoral dysfunction or patella alta. Any angle greater then 18° is often associated with patellofemoral dysfunction subluxing patella, increased femoral anteversion, genu valgum, or increased lateral tibial torsion.

## Glide Test

**Procedure:**  The patient is supine. The examiner stands at the patient's side next to the knee and grasps the proximal half of the patella with the thumb and index finger of one hand and the distal half with the thumb and index finger of the other. For the lateral glide test, the examiner's thumbs push the patella laterally over the lateral femoral condyle and the index fingers resting there. For the medial glide test, the examiner's index fingers push the patella in the opposite direction. In each case, the examiner's index finger or thumb can palpate the projecting posterior surface of the patella. Where increased lateral mobility is suspected, the same test is performed to assess stability with the quadriceps tensed. The patient is asked to lift his or her foot off the examining table. The examiner then notes the resulting motion of the patella. The medial and lateral glide test provides information about the degree of tension in the medial or lateral retinaculum, respectively. The test should always be performed comparatively on both knees.

With the hands in the same position, the examiner can also place traction on the patella by lifting it off the condyles.

**Assessment:**  Normal physiologic findings include symmetrical mobility of both patellae without any crepitation or tendency to dislocate. Increased lateral or medial mobility of the patella suggests laxity of the knee ligaments or habitual patellar subluxation or dislocation. Crepitation (retropatellar friction) occurring when the patella is mobilized suggests chondropathy or retropatellar osteoarthritis.

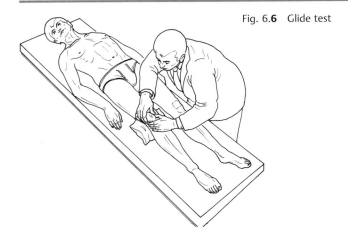

Fig. 6.**6**   Glide test

**Note:**   With the hands in the same position, the examiner can expand the test by moving the patella distally. Decreased distal mobility of the patella suggests shortening of the rectus femoris or patella alta.

### Zohlen Sign

**Procedure:**   The patient is supine with the leg extended. The examiner applies medial and lateral pressure to the proximal patella to press it into the trochlear groove and asks the patient to extend the leg further or tense the quadriceps. In the second phase, the examiner pushes down directly on the patella while the patient contracts the quadriceps. This test is called the Clarke sign or the patellar grind test.

**Assessment:**   The quadriceps exerts a proximal pull on the patella, pressing it tightly against the trochlear groove. This will cause retropatellar and/or peripatellar pain in the presence of retropatellar cartilage damage.

**Note:**   As this test, like the Zohlen sign, is often positive in normal patients, the best way is to repeat the procedure several times, increasing the pressure each time and comparing the results with those of the unaffected side. To test different parts of the patella, the knee should be tested in 30°, 60°, and 90° of flexion as well as in full extension.

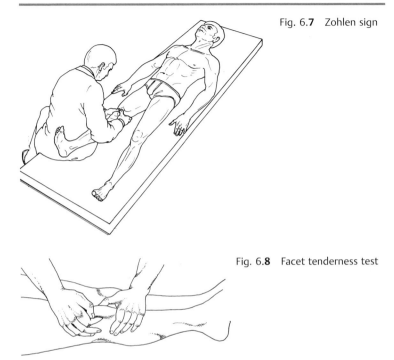

Fig. 6.**7**  Zohlen sign

Fig. 6.**8**  Facet tenderness test

## Facet Tenderness Test

**Procedure:**  The patient is supine with the knee extended. The examiner first elevates the medial margin of the patella with his or her thumbs and palpates the medial facet with a thumb, then elevates the lateral margin with the index fingers and palpates the lateral facet with an index finger. Elevating the patella allows palpation of the retropatellar region, which is important in disorders such as chondromalacia. Tenderness to palpation at the distal pole of the patella can be a sign of patellar tendinitis (*jumper's knee*).

**Assessment:**  Patients with retropatellar osteoarthritis, tendinitis, or synovitis will report pain, especially when the examiner palpates the medial facet.

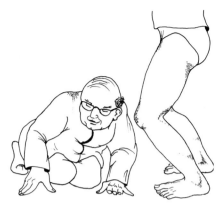

Fig. 6.**9**    Crepitation test

## Crepitation Test

**Procedure:**   The examiner kneels in front of the patient and asks the patient to crouch down or do a deep knee bend. The examiner listens for sounds posterior to the patella.

**Assessment:**   Crepitation ("snowball crunch" sound) suggests severe chondromalacia (grades II and III). Cracking sounds like those that occur in almost everyone during the first or second deep knee bend have no significance. For this reason, the patient is asked to do several deep knee bends. Usually the insignificant cracking sounds will decrease in intensity. In the absence of any audible retropatellar crepitation, the examiner may safely conclude that no severe retropatellar cartilage damage is present. However, the test results should not be used as a basis for far-reaching therapeutic decisions. They only provide information about the condition of the retropatellar cartilage. The crepitation test will be positive in many patients with normal knees.

## Fairbank Apprehension Test

**Procedure:**   The patient is supine with the knee extended and the thigh muscles relaxed. The examiner attempts to simulate a dislocation (in a manner similar to the apprehension test in anterior instability of the shoulder) by placing both thumbs on the medial aspect of the knee and pressing the patella laterally. The patient is asked to flex the knee.

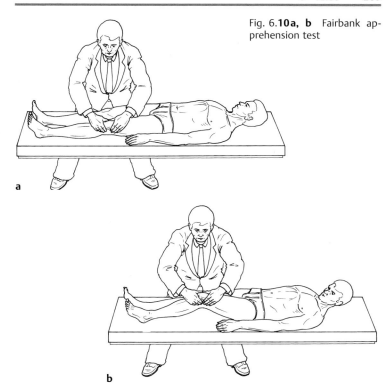

Fig. 6.**10a, b** Fairbank apprehension test

a

b

**Assessment:** Where a patella dislocation has occurred, the patient will report severe pain and will be apprehensive of another dislocation in extension or, at the latest, in flexion.

## McConnell Test

**Procedure:** The patient is seated with the legs relaxed and hanging over the edge of the table. This test attempts to provoke patellofemoral pain with isometric tensing of the quadriceps. This is done with the knee in various degrees of flexion (0°, 30°, 60°, and 120°). In each position, the examiner immobilizes the patient's lower leg and asks the patient to extend the leg against the examiner's resistance (this requires contraction of the quadriceps).

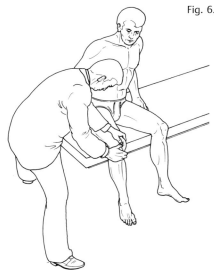

Fig. 6.**11**    McConnell test

**Assessment:**  Where the patient reports pain or a subjective sensation of constriction, the examiner medially displaces the patella with his or her thumb. In a positive test, this maneuver reduces pain. The examination should always be performed comparatively on both knees. Alleviation of pain by medial displacement of the patella is a diagnostic criterion for the presence of retropatellar pain.

**Note:**  In a positive McConnell test, pain can often be reduced by taping the knee so as to pull the patella medially. This "McConnell tape" bandage includes a lateral-to-medial slip that pulls the patella medially. A small plaster slip running medially from the middle of the patella is applied where a lateral patellar tilt requires correction. If required, a rotational slip extending from the medial knee to the tip of the patella and then to the lateral aspect can be applied to bring the patella into a neutral position. Physical therapy should concentrate on strengthening the vastus medialis and stretching the rectus femoris and iliotibial tract.

## Subluxation Suppression Test

Demonstrates lateral or medial patellar subluxation.

### Lateral Subluxation Suppression Test

**Procedure and assessment:**  To demonstrate lateral subluxation, the examiner places his or her thumbs on the proximal half of the lateral patellar facet. The patient is then asked to flex the knee. Either the thumb will be seen to prevent lateral subluxation or the examiner will feel the lateral motion of the patella. Flexing the knee without any attempt to prevent subluxation will lead to lateral patellar subluxation.

### Medial Subluxation Suppression Test

**Procedure and assessment:**  To demonstrate medial subluxation, the examiner places his or her index fingers on the proximal half of the medial patellar facet. The patient is then asked to flex the knee. The examiner's finger will be seen to prevent medial subluxation. In contrast, flexing the knee without any attempt to prevent subluxation will lead to medial patellar subluxation (this is extremely rare).

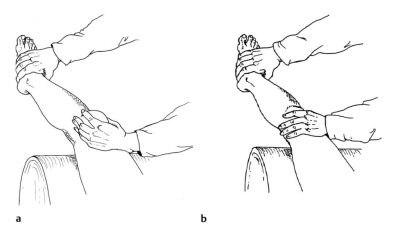

a                                            b

Fig. 6.**12a, b**   Subluxation suppression test:
**a** lateral subluxation test,
**b** medial subluxation test

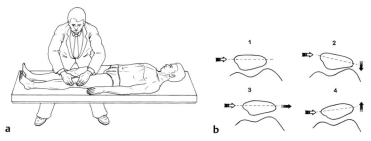

Fig. 6.**13a, b**   Tilt test:
**a**  passive lateralization of the patella;
**b**  starting position (*1*), negative "abnormal" tilt test (*2*), neutral test (*3*), positive test (*4*)

## Tilt Test

**Procedure:**   The patient is supine. The examiner passively displaces the patella laterally, noting how it behaves during lateral displacement.

**Assessment:**   Where the lateral retinaculum is very tight due to contracture, the lateral facet will dip toward the femur (negative "abnormal" tilt test). Where there is normal tone in the retinaculum, the patella will remain at roughly the same height with respect to the femur (neutral tilt test). With laxity of the lateral retinaculum and with generalized ligament laxity, the lateral margin of the patella will rise up out of the trochlear groove (positive tilt test).

**Note:**   The primary purpose of the tilt test is to evaluate tension in the lateral retinaculum. Where the tilt test is neutral or positive, a lateral release to decompress the patellofemoral joint will hardly improve symptoms at all. However, it may be expected to improve symptoms in cases where the tilt test is negative. Patients with a positive tilt test greater than 5° and medial and lateral gliding of the patella exhibit poor results after an isolated lateral release. Dysplasia of the trochlear groove can lead to atypical test results. The tilt test should always be performed comparatively on both knees.

## Mediopatellar Plica Test

**Procedure:** The patient lies in the supine position and the examiner flexes the affected knee to 30°.

**Assessment:** If the examiner then moves the patella medially, the patient complains of pain. This pain, indicating a positive test, is caused by pinching of the edge of the plica between the medial condyle and the patella. The pain may be indicative of a mediopatellar plica.

## Hughston Plica Test

**Procedure:** The patient lies in the supine position and the examiner flexes the knee and medially rotates the tibia with one arm and hand while pressing the patella medially with the heel of the other hand and palpating the medial femoral condyle with the fingers of the same hand. The patient's knee is passively flexed and extended while the examiner feels for "popping" of the plical band under the fingers.

**Assessment:** The popping indicates a positive test for a mediopatellar plica syndrome.

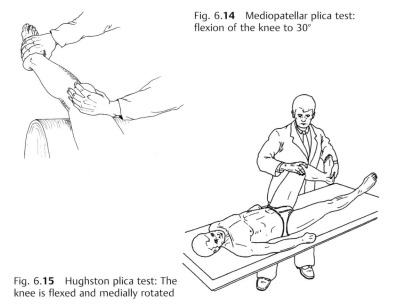

Fig. 6.**14** Mediopatellar plica test: flexion of the knee to 30°

Fig. 6.**15** Hughston plica test: The knee is flexed and medially rotated

**Dreyer Test**

Assesses a quadriceps tendon tear at the superior pole of the patella.

**Procedure:**  The supine patient is asked to raise the extended leg. If the patient is unable to do so, the examiner stabilizes the quadriceps tendon proximal to the patella and has the patient lift the leg again.

**Assessment:**  When stabilizing the tendon allows the patient to lift the leg, the examiner should suspect an avulsion of the quadriceps tendon from the patella or a chronic patellar fracture in applicable cases.

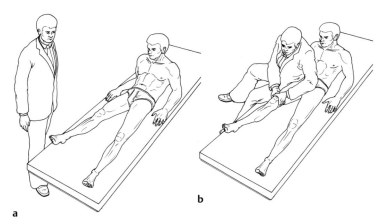

**b**

**a**

Fig. 6.**16a, b**    Dreyer test:
**a** abnormal: patient is unable to lift the leg;
**b** with the examiner stabilizing the patella

## ■ Meniscus

The menisci are important in guiding motion and ensuring stability in the knee. They also transmit and distribute compressive stresses between the femur and tibia. Meniscus injuries include tears or avulsions of the cartilage disks. Anatomic factors predispose the medial meniscus to a far higher incidence of injury than the lateral meniscus.

Meniscus lesions be degenerative or traumatic in origin. Degenerative meniscus conditions usually first manifest themselves as increasing pain with exercise. Usually a minor injury will suffice to produce a tear in a weakened meniscus. In diagnosing knee injuries, one must always be alert to the possibility of a combined injury involving the collateral and cruciate ligaments in addition to the meniscus injury. Any insufficiently treated ligament injury with instability of the knee can also lead to meniscus damage. The primary symptoms of late sequelae of meniscus injuries include pain with exercise accompanied by occasional impingement symptoms and joint effusions with irritation.

There are a number of diagnostic signs of meniscus damage. The function tests are based on pain provocation as a result of compression, traction, or shear forces acting on the meniscus.

An isolated function test will rarely be sufficient to evaluate a meniscus lesion. Usually a combination of various maneuvers is required to confirm the diagnosis.

## Apley Distraction and Compression Test (Grinding Test)

**Procedure:**  The patient is prone with the affected knee flexed 90°. The examiner immobilizes the patient's thigh with his or her knee. In this position, the examiner rotates the patient's knee while alternately applying axial traction and compression to the lower leg.

**Assessment:**  Pain in the flexed knee occurring during rotation of the lower leg with traction applied suggests injury to the capsular ligaments (positive distraction test). Pain with compression applied suggests a meniscus lesion (positive grinding test).

Snapping phenomena can occur with discoid menisci or meniscal cysts. Pain in internal rotation suggests injury to the lateral meniscus or lateral capsule and/or ligaments; pain in external rotation suggests injury to the medial meniscus or medial capsule and/or ligaments.

The sign cannot be elicited where the capsular ligaments are tight, nor is this possible in an injury to the posterior horn of the lateral meniscus.

Wirth describes a modification of the grinding test (compression test), in which the knee is extended with the lower leg in fixed rotation. Wirth was able to confirm the presence of a meniscus lesion in over 85% of all cases with this modified Apley test.

## McMurray Test (Fouche Sign)

**Procedure:**  The patient is supine with the knee and hip of the affected leg in maximum flexion. The examiner grasps the patient's knee with one hand and the patient's foot with the other. Holding the patient's lower leg in maximum external or internal rotation, the examiner then passively extends the knee into 90° of flexion.

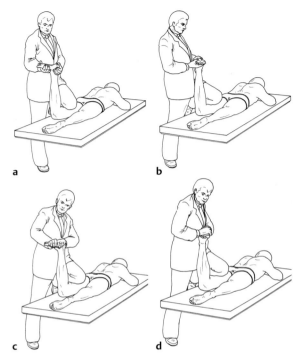

Fig. 6.**17 a–d**   Apley distraction and compression test:
**a** distraction and external rotation,
**b** distraction and internal rotation,
**c** compression and external rotation,
**d** compression and internal rotation

**Assessment:**   Pain while extending the knee with the lower leg externally rotated and abducted suggests a medial meniscus lesion; pain in internal rotation suggests an injury to the lateral meniscus. A snapping sound in extreme flexion occurs when a projecting meniscal flap becomes impinged on the posterior horn. Snapping in 90° of flexion suggests an injury in the middle section of the meniscus.

The snapping symptoms can be increased by moving the entire lower leg in a circle (modified McMurray test).

**Note:**   Continuing the extension as far as the neutral (0°) position corresponds to the Bragard test. This test, when performed by slowly extending the knee with the lower leg in internal rotation, is also

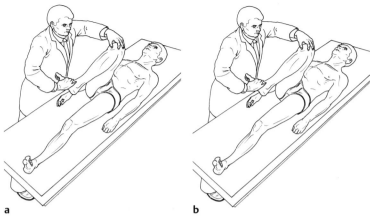

Fig. 6.**18a, b**   McMurray test:
**a** in maximum flexion,
**b** in 90° of flexion

described as the Fouche sign. The McMurray test is positive in 30% of all children with normal knees. Approximately 1% of the normal population should test positive.

### Bragard Test

**Procedure:**   The patient is supine. With one hand, the examiner grasps the patient's 90°-flexed knee and palpates the lateral and medial joint cavity with the thumb and index finger. With the other hand, the examiner grasps the patient's foot and rotates the patient's lower leg.

**Assessment:**   Pain felt over the joint cavity indicates a meniscus lesion. In an injury to the medial meniscus, external rotation and extension from a flexed position increases the pain in the medial joint cavity.

   With internal rotation and increasing flexion in the knee, the meniscus migrates back into the interior of the joint and is no longer accessible to the examiner's palpating finger. This reduces pain.

   Where a lateral meniscus lesion is suspected, the examiner palpates the lateral meniscus. This is done while first extending and internally rotating the knee from a position of maximum flexion. Pain in the lateral joint space is a sign of lateral meniscus injury. In external rotation and increasing flexion, the meniscus shifts back into the interior of the joint and is no longer palpable with the finger. This maneuver reduces pain.

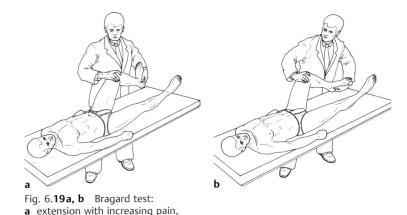

Fig. 6.**19a, b**   Bragard test:
**a** extension with increasing pain,
**b** migrating tenderness to palpation

The diagnosis is more certain if the tenderness to palpation migrates with joint motions. The lateral meniscus, and with it the tenderness to palpation, migrates posteriorly as the knee is internally rotated.

### Payr Sign

**Procedure:**   The patient is seated cross-legged. The examiner exerts intermittent pressure on the affected leg, which is flexed and externally rotated.

**Assessment:**   Pain in the medial joint cavity suggests meniscus damage (usually a lesion of the posterior horn). Occasionally, patients themselves will be able to provoke snapping. Moving the knee back and forth causes the injured portion of the meniscus to be drawn into the joint and then spring back out with a snap when the joint cavity is distended.

### Payr Test

**Procedure:**   The patient is supine. The examiner immobilizes the patient's knee with his or her left hand and palpates the lateral and medial joint cavity with the thumb and index finger, respectively. With the other hand, the examiner grasps the patient's ankle. With the knee maximally flexed, the lower leg is externally rotated as far as possible.

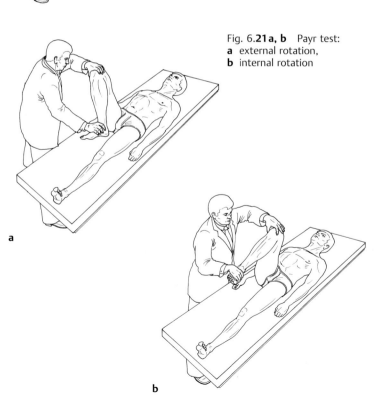

Fig. 6.**20** Payr sign

Fig. 6.**21a, b** Payr test:
**a** external rotation,
**b** internal rotation

a

b

Then with the knee in slight adduction (varus stress), the leg is flexed further in the direction of the contralateral hip.

**Assessment:**   Pain in the posterior medial joint cavity suggests damage to the medial meniscus (most often the posterior horn is involved, which is compressed by this maneuver). The posterior horn of the lateral meniscus can be similarly examined with the knee internally rotated and abducted (valgus stress).

### Steinmann I Sign

**Procedure:**   The patient is supine. The examiner immobilizes the patient's flexed knee with the left hand and grasps the lower leg with the other hand. The examiner then forcefully rotates the lower leg in various degrees of knee flexion.

**Assessment:**   Pain in the medial joint cavity in forced external rotation suggests damage to the medial meniscus; pain in the lateral joint cavity

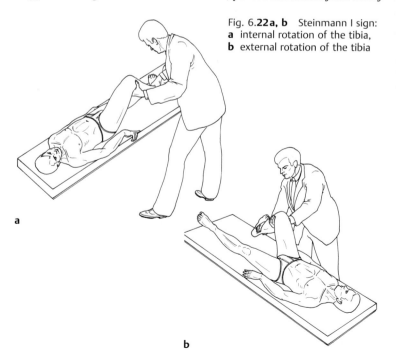

Fig. 6.**22a, b**   Steinmann I sign:
**a** internal rotation of the tibia,
**b** external rotation of the tibia

in internal rotation suggests damage to the lateral meniscus. Because the localization of the tear can vary, the test for the Steinmann I sign should be performed with the knee in varying degrees of flexion.

## Steinmann II Sign

**Procedure:** The patient is supine. The examiner grasps the knee with the left hand and palpates the joint cavity. With the right hand, the examiner grasps the patient's lower leg slightly proximal to the mortise of the ankle. With the patient's thigh immobilized, the examiner places

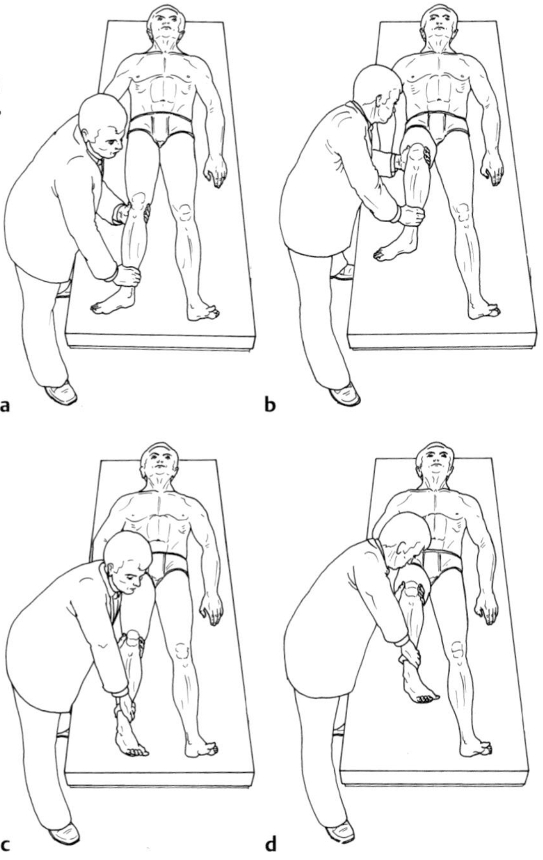

Fig. 6.**23a–d**
Steinmann II sign:
**a** starting position with the lower leg externally rotated,
**b** flexion,
**c** starting position with the lower leg internally rotated,
**d** flexion

a

b

c

d

the lower leg first in external rotation, then in internal rotation, in each case alternately flexing and extending the lower leg while applying slight axial compression.

**Assessment:**   Pain in the medial or lateral joint cavity suggests a meniscus injury. The tenderness to palpation in the joint cavity migrates medially and posteriorly during flexion and slight external rotation of the knee; it then migrates back anteriorly as the knee is extended. Where a meniscus injury is suspected and the lower leg is placed in internal rotation, the tenderness to palpation will migrate anteriorly as the knee is extended and posteriorly as it is flexed.

**Note:**   Although this test can also be used for an injury to the lateral meniscus, its primary purpose is to help evaluate medial meniscus lesions. A differential diagnosis must consider osteoarthritis and lesions of the medial collateral and capsular ligaments.

### Boehler–Kroemer Test

**Procedure:**   The patient is supine. The examiner stabilizes the lateral femur with one hand and grasps the medial malleolus with the other. With the lower leg abducted (valgus stress applied), the examiner then passively flexes and extends the knee.

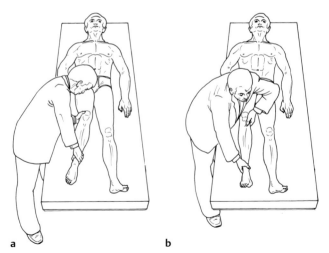

**a**                          **b**

Fig. 6.**24a, b**   Boehler–Kroemer test:
**a** lower leg abducted (valgus), **b** lower leg adducted (varus)

With his or her hands on the patient's lateral malleolus and medial thigh, the examiner grasps the leg and flexes and extends the knee with the lower leg adducted (varus stress applied).

**Assessment:** Flexing and extending the knee with the lower leg alternately adducted and abducted (the Kroemer test) alternately increases compression of the medial meniscus and lateral meniscus. Opening the joint cavity compresses the opposite meniscus. Opening the medial cavity creates a valgus stress for testing the lateral meniscus; opening the lateral cavity creates a varus stress for testing the medial meniscus.

**Note:** The Boehler meniscus tests in the coronal plane (with the knee extended) allow simultaneous assessment of the ligaments of the knee in the side opposite the motion.

### Merke Test

**Procedure:** The patient bears weight on the affected leg with the knee slightly flexed. The examiner immobilizes the foot of the affected leg.
The examiner lifts the patient's contralateral leg slightly and asks the patient to internally and externally rotate the thigh of the affected leg.
The lower leg is rotated as in the Steinmann I test.

**Assessment:** Because of the increased axial compression due to the weight of the body, the Merke test usually elicits more severe pain. Pain occurring in the medial joint cavity in internal rotation of the thigh (corresponding to external rotation of the lower leg) suggests a medial meniscus lesion.
Pain occurring in external rotation of the thigh (corresponding to internal rotation of the lower leg) suggests a lateral meniscus lesion.
The Merke test is occasionally positive in the presence of collateral ligament lesions.

### Cabot Test

**Procedure:** The patient is supine with the affected leg flexed at the knee and placed over the proximal portion of the contralateral lower leg. With his or her left hand, the examiner grasps the patient's knee and palpates the lateral joint cavity with the thumb. With the other hand, the examiner grasps the patient's lower leg slightly proximal to the subtalar joint. The patient is then asked to extend the knee against the resistance of the examiner's hand.

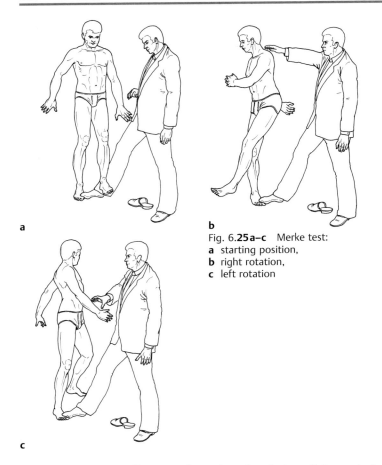

**a**

**b**

Fig. 6.**25 a–c**  Merke test:
**a**  starting position,
**b**  right rotation,
**c**  left rotation

**c**

**Assessment:**   Pain will occur where there is a lesion of the posterior horn of the lateral meniscus. Depending on the severity of the pain, the patient will often be unable to extend the knee farther. The painful point, which palpable with the thumb, lies primarily in the lateral posterior joint cavity. Occasionally patients will report pain radiating into the popliteal fossa and calf.

**Note:**   The Cabot test is also described in the literature as the popliteus sign.

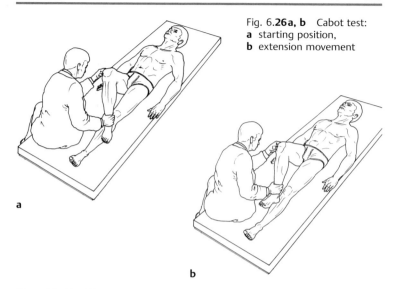

Fig. 6.**26a, b** Cabot test:
**a** starting position,
**b** extension movement

**a**

**b**

## Finochietto Sign

Simultaneously tests cruciate ligament and meniscus injuries.

**Procedure:** The patient is supine. The anterior drawer test is performed with the knee flexed 90°.

**Assessment:** Where the injury also involves an anterior cruciate ligament tear, the anterior drawer test with the knee flexed 90° will cause anterior displacement of the tibia. The laxity of the knee ligaments causes the femoral condyle to ride up over the posterior horn of the medial meniscus under the stress of the anterior drawer. A positive Finochietto test produces an audible snap and/or a palpable skip. If the tibia is then pressed posteriorly, the femoral condyle will glide back down from the posterior horn of the medial meniscus. Occasionally, reduction of the displaced meniscus will be necessary following a positive Finochietto test. In this case, there is reason to suspect a full posterior separation of the medial meniscus and/or a longitudinal or bucket handle tear.

**Note:** In the setting of anterior cruciate ligament insufficiency, damage to the posterior horn of the medial meniscus or its capsular attachments results from derangement of the rolling and sliding mechanism secondary to a cruciate ligament tear. This produces a shear injury to the posterior horn of the medial meniscus.

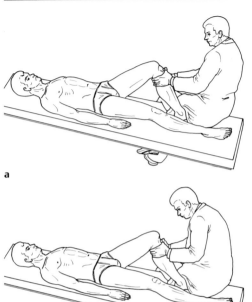

Fig. 6.**27a, b** Finochietto sign:
**a** anterior drawer,
**b** reduction

## Childress Sign

**Procedure:**   The patient assumes a squatting position, preferably with the buttocks in contact with the heels. The patient is then asked to waddle in this position.

**Assessment:**   In the presence of an injury to the posterior horn, the patient will notice a painful snapping shortly before maximum flexion or in the early phase of extension. This is caused by impingement of the injured meniscus. Patients in severe pain will usually be unable to assume the squatting position.

## Turner Sign

In 1931, Turner described a meniscus sign caused by chronic irritation of the infrapatellar branch of the saphenous nerve. A meniscus lesion will often be accompanied by an irregular hyperesthetic area measuring

Fig. 6.**28** Childress sign

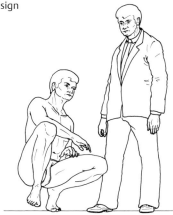

approximately 4–5 cm. This area will be located at the level of and slightly proximal to the medial joint cavity on the medial aspect of the knee or along the course of the infrapatellar branch of the saphenous nerve. Thermal and mechanical stimuli (tapping) are used to test the area for local hypersensitivity. According to Zippel, careful examination technique will demonstrate this symptom more often than one would expect. No similar sign is known for injuries to the lateral meniscus.

## Anderson Medial and Lateral Compression Test

**Procedure:** The patient is supine. The examiner grasps the patient's lower leg and immobilizes the foot between his or her own forearm and waist. With the free hand, the examiner palpates the anterior joint cavity. The examiner the flexes the knee to 45° while applying a valgus stress and extends it while applying a varus stress. This produces a circular movement in the knee.

**Assessment:** A longitudinal or flap tear in the meniscus causes pain and/or friction rub at the level of the joint cavity. Complex tears lead to chronic friction rub. However, the same symptoms can occur with osteoarthritis or secondary to resection of a meniscus. This test involves placing stresses on the knee as it approaches extension and in moderate flexion. Therefore, one can occasionally provoke subluxation as the knee approaches extension as in a positive pivot shift test with insufficiency of the anterior cruciate ligament.

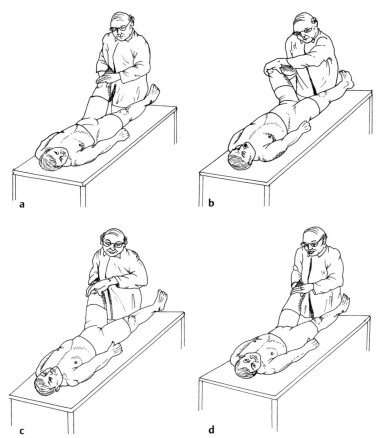

Fig. 6.**29a–d**   Anderson medial and lateral compression test:
**a** starting position,
**b** valgus stress during flexion of the knee to 45°,
**c** extension of the 45° flexed knee,
**d** varus stress during extension of the knee

## Paessler Rotational Compression Test

**Procedure:**   The patient is seated. The examiner immobilizes the foot of the leg to be examined, holding it between his or her own legs slightly proximal to the knees. To evaluate the medial meniscus, the examiner

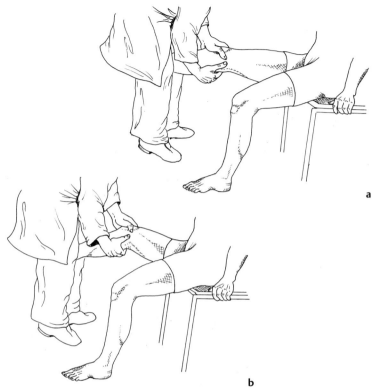

Fig. 6.**30a, b**   Paessler rotational compression test:
**a** starting position with examiner's thumb on medial joint cavity,
**b** circular motion of the knee

rests both thumbs on the medial joint cavity and moves the patient's knee in a circle in the form of external and internal rotational movements. This causes the knee to move through various degrees of flexion. At the same time, the examiner applies a varus or valgus stress, respectively.

**Assessment:**   The test is positive when the patient reports pain with the circular motion. It is considered strongly positive when pain can be elicited by the circular motion alone in either the medial joint cavity (suspected lateral meniscus lesion) or the lateral joint cavity (suspected medial meniscus lesion).

## Tschaklin Sign

Quadriceps atrophy is often encountered in chronic meniscus lesions. Atrophy of the vastus medialis in medial meniscus lesions is often associated with compensatory increase in muscle tone in the sartorius, which is known as the Tschaklin sign.

## Wilson Test

### Indicates Osteochondritis Dissecans

**Procedure:** The patient lies in a supine position with the knee flexed to 90°. The patient actively extends the knee while maintaining the tibia in internal rotation. The patient is told to stop the motion and hold the knee in the position in which pain is experienced. If pain is experienced, the patient is instructed to externally rotate the tibia while the knee is held at its present point of flexion.

**Assessment:** The test is positive if pain experienced during extension with internal tibial rotation is relieved by externally rotating the tibia. The lesion of the knee is at the classic site of osteochondritis dissecans of the medial femoral condyle near the intercondylar fossa.

**Note:** Osteochondritis dissecans is an aseptic necrosis that arises in the subchondral bone of the articular surfaces and disrupts the overlying cartilage. In its advanced stages, separation of part of the articular cartilage and underlying bone can occur, creating an intraarticular loose body. Osteochondritis dissecans should always be considered in adolescents presenting with joint effusion and knee pain.

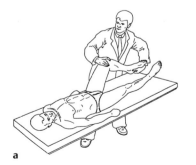
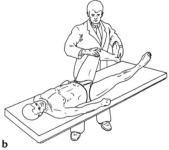

a    b

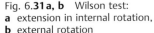

Fig. 6.**31 a, b**   Wilson test:
**a** extension in internal rotation,
**b** external rotation

# ■ Knee Ligament Stability Tests

The knee is stabilized by the ligaments, menisci, the shape and congruency of the articular surfaces, and the musculature. The ligaments ensure functional congruency by guiding the femur and tibia and limiting the space between them. Ligament injuries lead to functional impairment of the knee with instability. Knee ligament stability tests can help to identify and differentiate these instabilities.

Abnormal directions of motion can be divided into three categories:

1. Direct instability in a single plane
2. Rotational instability
3. Combined rotational instability

Clinical instability is divided into three degrees. Estimated joint opening or drawer of up to 5 mm is defined as 1+ (or +), 5–10 mm as 2+ (++), and over 10 mm as 3+ (or +++).

## Abduction and Adduction Test (Valgus and Varus Stress Test)

Assesses medial and lateral knee stability.

**Procedure:**   The patient is supine. The examiner grasps the patient's knee at the tibial head with both hands while palpating the joint cavity. The examiner immobilizes the patient's distal lower leg between his or her own forearm and waist while applying a valgus and varus stress to the knee. The fingers resting on the joint cavity can palpate any opening of the joint.

**Assessment:**   Lateral stability is assessed in 20° of flexion and in full extension. Full extension prevents lateral opening as long as the posterior capsule and posterior cruciate ligament are intact, even if the medial collateral ligament is torn. In 20° of flexion, the posterior capsule is relaxed. Applying a valgus stress in this position evaluates the medial collateral ligament alone as the primary stabilizer. This allows the examiner to identify the nature of damage to the posteromedial capsular ligaments.

The opposite applies to adduction (varus) stress. In 20° of flexion, the primary lateral stabilizer is the lateral collateral ligament. The anterior cruciate ligament and popliteus tendon act as secondary stabilizers.

When testing lateral stability, the examiner assessed the degree of joint opening and the quality of the endpoint.

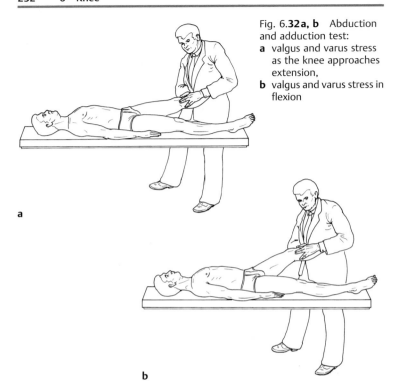

Fig. 6.**32a, b**   Abduction and adduction test:
**a** valgus and varus stress as the knee approaches extension,
**b** valgus and varus stress in flexion

a

b

## ◼ Function Tests to Assess the Anterior Cruciate Ligament

### Lachman Test

**Procedure:**   The patient is supine. The examiner holds the patient's knee between 15° and 30° of flexion.

In this position in particular, the stabilizing function of the anterior cruciate ligament is essential in changing direction and braking. In these positions of the knee as it approaches extension, insufficiency of the anterior cruciate will be observable as lateral subluxation of the proximal tibia (pivoting).

The tibia should be slightly laterally rotated and the anterior tibial translation force should be applied from the posteromedial aspect.

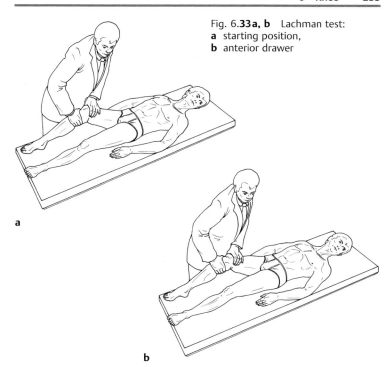

Fig. 6.**33a, b** Lachman test:
**a** starting position,
**b** anterior drawer

a

b

**Assessment:** The anterior cruciate ligament is damaged when mobility of the tibia with respect to the femur can be demonstrated. The end-point of motion must be soft and gradual without a hard stop; any hard stop suggests a certain stability of the anterior cruciate ligament. A hard endpoint within 3 mm suggests complete stability of the anterior cruciate, whereas one after 5 mm or more suggests relative stability of the anterior cruciate ligament, such as may be present following an earlier sprain.

Cruciate ligament injury should be suspected where the endpoint is soft or absent. In the presence of a drawer exceeding 5 mm, comparison with the contralateral knee is helpful in excluding congenital laxity of the articular ligaments.

A positive Lachman test is certain proof of anterior cruciate ligament insufficiency. A false-negative test may occur if the femur is not properly stabilized, if a meniscus lesion or degenerative changes such as osteo-phytes on the intercondylar eminence block translation, or if the tibia is medially rotated.

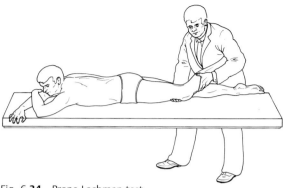

Fig. 6.**34**    Prone Lachman test

## Prone Lachman Test

**Procedure:**   The patient is prone. The examiner grasps the lateral aspect of the proximal tibia and immobilizes the patient's leg in his or her own axilla. With the other hand, the examiner grasps the distal femur immediately proximal to the patella to immobilize the thigh. Then the examiner pushes the tibia anteriorly with respect to the femur.

**Assessment:**   Damage to the cruciate ligament is present where there is demonstrable mobility of the tibia relative to the femur. The motion must have a soft endpoint. Any hard endpoint suggests a certain stability of the anterior cruciate. Where this occurs within 3 mm, it suggests complete stability; where it only occurs after 5 mm, it suggests relative stability with previous elongation of the anterior cruciate.

Cruciate ligament injury should be assumed where the endpoint is soft or absent. In drawer motion exceeding 5 mm, comparison with the contralateral side is helpful in excluding congenital laxity of the articular ligaments.

A positive Lachman test is proof of insufficiency of the anterior cruciate ligament.

**Note:**   Although the patient is relaxed in the prone position, it is not always easy to assess the quality of the endpoint. A hard endpoint and hemarthrosis suggest an acute partial tear; a hard endpoint without hemarthrosis suggests a suspected chronic partial tear, elongation, or excessive laxity.

A soft endpoint and hemarthrosis suggest a complete tear; a soft endpoint without hemarthrosis suggests a chronic complete tear.

Fig. 6.**35** Stable Lachman test

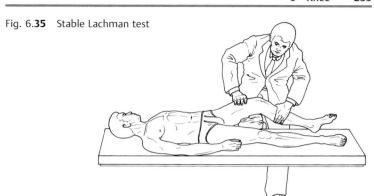

Where the endpoint is hard, a posterior cruciate lesion must be excluded by testing the spontaneous posterior drawer and applying the active tests.

## Stable Lachman Test

A variation of the classic Lachman test.

**Procedure:** The patient is supine. The examiner places the patient's thigh over his or her own thigh. This holds the patient's leg in constant flexion that the patient cannot change. With the distal hand, the examiner pulls the tibia anteriorly while the other hand immobilizes the patient's thigh on the examiner's own thigh.

**Assessment:** Identical to the classic Lachman test.

**Note:** The classic Lachman test not only presents problems for examiners with small hands; simultaneously immobilizing the thigh and lower leg can be also difficult for any examiner with an obese or muscular patient. Using one's own thigh as a "workbench" for examining the patient's knee is an easy solution in such cases and one that allows examination even of obese or muscular patients. The character of the endpoint (hard or soft) is easier to evaluate in this test.

## No-Touch Lachman Test

**Procedure:** The patient is supine and grasps the thigh of the affected leg near the knee with both hands and slightly flexes the knee. The patient is then asked to raise the lower leg off the examining table while

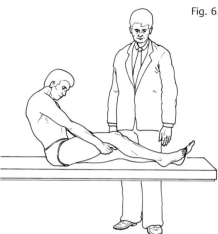

Fig. 6.**36**   No-touch Lachman test

maintaining flexion in the knee. The examiner observes the position of the tibial tuberosity during this maneuver.

**Assessment:**   If the ligaments are intact, there will be no change in contour, or only a slight one as the tibial tuberosity moves slightly anteriorly. In an acute injury to the capsular ligaments involving the anterior cruciate and medial collateral ligaments, the examiner will observe a significant anterior displacement of the tibial tuberosity (subluxation of the joint).

**Note:**   This test often allows one to exclude complex injuries without having to touch the patient.

### Active Lachman Test

**Procedure:**   The examiner asks the supine patient to extend the leg in such as way as to lift the foot off the examining table. During this maneuver, the examiner keeps his or her eyes on the knee the better to discern the contours of the tibial tuberosity and patellar ligament. The examiner achieves slight passive flexion in the knee by passing one hand beneath the thigh of the patient's affected leg and resting it on the contralateral knee. The effect of the quadriceps is increased by immobilizing the foot on the examining table.

**Assessment:**   Slight migration of the tibial head will be observed where the anterior cruciate ligament is intact. In a cruciate tear, there will be a

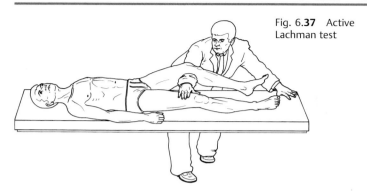

Fig. 6.**37**   Active Lachman test

significant anterior migration compared with the contralateral side. This is because the anterior cruciate ligament no longer limits the displacement caused by contraction of the quadriceps.

**Note:**   The physiologic drawer in active motion as the knee approaches extension usually measures 2–3 mm. In contrast, tibial displacement of 3–6 mm will be observed with an anterior cruciate ligament tear. This test should only be performed after excluding a posterior cruciate ligament injury, in which the tibia would spontaneously displace posteriorly. There, too, contraction of the quadriceps will produce significant anterior displacement of the tibia and with it a false-positive active anterior drawer test.

Contraction of the quadriceps can also cause meniscal impingement where loosening of the posterior attachment of the medial meniscus accompanies the insufficiency of the medial ligaments and anterior cruciate.

The active Lachman test differs from the traditional Lachman test in that the lower leg can easily be immobilized in various degrees of rotation and the stabilizing effect of the medial and lateral capsular ligaments can be assessed. Generalized anterior instability (involving the anterior cruciate ligament and the medial, posteromedial, lateral, and posterolateral capsular ligaments) will produce significant active anterior tibial displacement in internal and neutral rotation and, especially, in external rotation.

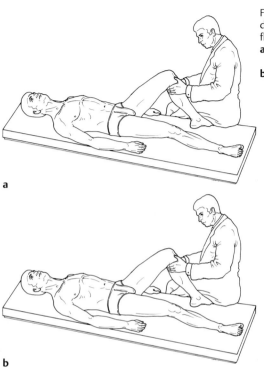

Fig. 6.**38a, b**   Anterior drawer test in 90° flexion:
**a**  starting position in external rotation,
**b**  anterior traction on the tibia

a

b

## Anterior Drawer Test in 90° Flexion

Passive anterior drawer test to assess the stability of the anterior cruciate ligament.

**Procedure:**  The patient is supine with the hip flexed 45° and the knee flexed 90°. The examiner sits on the edge of the examining table and uses his or her buttocks to immobilize the patient's foot in the desired rotational position. The examiner then grasps the tibial head with both hands and pulls it anteriorly with the patient's knee flexors relaxed. The test is performed in a neutral position, with the foot in 15° of external rotation to assess anterior and medial instability, and with the foot in 30° of internal rotation to assess anterior and lateral instability.

**Assessment:**  A visible and palpable anterior drawer (that is, anterior displacement of the tibia with a soft endpoint) is present in chronic insufficiency of the anterior cruciate ligament.

The anterior drawer test in 90° of flexion is often negative in acute injuries because pain often prevents the patient from achieving this degree of flexion and causes reflexive muscle contraction. Additionally, these are usually combined injuries involving complete or partial ligament tears so that the stress of the drawer test stretches the partially torn medial and lateral structures. The resulting pain produces false-negative test results, giving the appearance of a stable joint.

In acute injuries in particular, the test should preferably be performed with the knee in slight flexion (Lachman test). The situation is different in chronic ligament injuries, where the primary symptom is the sensation of instability. In these cases, the test can usually be performed painlessly in 90° of flexion and still provide useful diagnostic information.

**Note:** As a rule, the anterior drawer is best assessed in neutral rotation. This allows one to demonstrate the greatest degree of displacement. Rotation forces the tibia into a position where the twisting of the peripheral ligaments and capsular structures increases tension in the joint, impairing the mobility of the drawer. Assessment of rotational stability together with assessment of lateral stability in flexion and extension provides information about the complexity of the ligament injury and the stability of the secondary stabilizers.

An anterior drawer should not automatically be interpreted as an anterior cruciate ligament tear. On the other hand, a negative drawer test does not necessarily confirm that the anterior cruciate is intact. The proximal portion of the tibia is pulled anteriorly or pushed posteriorly. It can be difficult to determine the exact starting position (the neutral position) from which an anteriorly directed force will produce an anterior drawer. For example, where the examiner exerts an anterior drawer stress in the presence of a posterior cruciate ligament injury in which the tibial head is posteriorly depressed (a spontaneous posterior drawer), it will seem as if an isolated anterior drawer were present. What has actually happened in this case is that the tibia has merely been drawn anteriorly out of its posterior displacement (due to the posterior cruciate tear) and into a neutral position. The anterior cruciate then tenses and limits further anterior displacement of the tibia.

**Caution:** An apparent anterior drawer may only be interpreted as a true anterior drawer once the absence of a posterior drawer has been demonstrated.

## Jakob Maximum Drawer Test

**Procedure:**  The patient is supine with the knee flexed 50°–60°. The examiner pushes the tibial head into maximum anterior subluxation with his or her forearm while grasping the patient's contralateral knee with the hand of the same arm. With the other hand, the examiner grasps the tibial head and palpates how far anteriorly the medial or

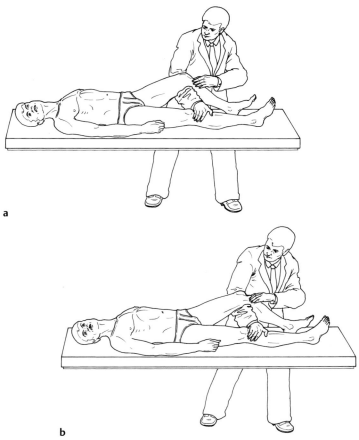

**a**

**b**

Fig. 6.**39a, b**  Jakob maximum drawer test:
**a** starting position,
**b** maximum anterior traction on the tibia

lateral joint cavity is displaced. The patient's lower leg is not immobilized in this test so that rotation is not restricted. This allows maximum tibial displacement.

**Assessment:**  See anterior drawer test in 90° flexion.

## Pivot Shift Test

**Procedure:**  The patient is supine. The examiner grasps and immobilizes the lateral femoral condyle with one hand and palpates the proximal tibia or fibula with the thumb. With the other hand, the examiner

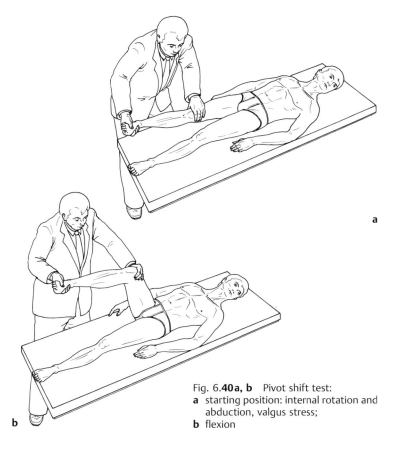

Fig. 6.**40a, b**  Pivot shift test:
**a** starting position: internal rotation and abduction, valgus stress;
**b** flexion

holds the patient's lower leg in internal rotation and abduction (valgus stress). From this starting position the knee is then moved from extension into flexion.

**Assessment:**  In the presence of a torn anterior cruciate ligament, the valgus stress will cause the tibia to subluxate anteriorly while the knee is still in extension. The blockade of the knee in anterior subluxation depends on the degree of valgus stress applied; occasionally the sign can be elicited more easily when the examiner immobilizes the patient's leg between his or her own forearm and waist while applying slight axial compression. The knee is then flexed while the same internal rotation and abduction of the lower leg is maintained; this then causes the subluxated tibial head to reduce posteriorly at 20°–40° of flexion. The iliotibial tract, which with increasing flexion glides from a position anterior to the lateral epicondyle in extension to a position posterior to the axis of flexion, draws the tibial head posteriorly again. The degree of reduction and flexion depends on the severity of the anterior subluxation. Reduction occurs earlier when there is only slight anterior translation. The patient usually confirms the diagnosis by reporting that the typical sensation of the knee giving way felt in sports activities can be reproduced in this test.

According to Jakob, a genuine pivot shift phenomenon can partially disappear, despite anterior cruciate ligament insufficiency, under the following conditions:

1. When a complete tear of the medial collateral ligament is present, the valgus opening prevents force concentration in the lateral compartment. Subluxation cannot occur under these circumstances.
2. When the iliotibial tract is traumatically divided, only the subluxation will be observed, not the abrupt reduction.
3. A bucket handle tear of the medial or lateral meniscus can prevent anterior translation or reduction of the tibia.
4. Increasing osteoarthritis in the lateral compartment with osteophytes can create a concave contour along the once convex lateral tibial plateau.

## Jakob Graded Pivot Shift Test

Gradation of the pivot shift test allowing for translation and rotation of the tibia.

**Procedure:**  The procedure is identical to the pivot shift test except that here instability of the knee is assessed with the lower leg in not only internal rotation, but in neutral and external rotation as well.

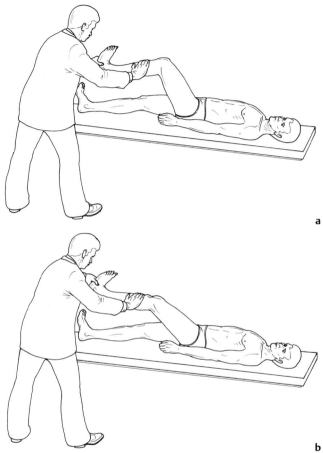

Fig. 6.**41 a, b**   Jakob graded pivot shift test:
**a** starting position: flexion and internal rotation of lower leg, valgus stress on the knee;
**b** anterior subluxation of the lateral tibial head as the knee approaches extension with lower leg internally rotated and valgus stress on the knee

**Assessment:**   Pivot shift grade I: The pivot shift test is positive only in maximum internal rotation; it is negative in neutral and internal rotation. The subluxation as the knee approaches extension is more palpable than visible to the examiner (slight translation may be apparent).

Pivot shift grade II: The pivot shift test is positive in internal and neutral rotation; however, it is negative in external rotation. There is visible and palpable translation on the lateral aspect of the joint.

Pivot shift grade III: The pivot shift test is clearly positive in neutral rotation and particularly conspicuous in external rotation. The sign is less distinct in internal rotation.

Pivot shift grade IV can only be demonstrated in acute knee injuries where the posteromedial and lateral structures are damaged in addition to the anterior cruciate. In chronic instability, a grade III pivot shift will be detectable in cases where the secondary stabilizers have loosened over time.

**Note:**    In an anterior cruciate tear, both the medial and lateral portions of the tibia migrate anteriorly under the stress of the anterior drawer.

In an isolated tear of the anterior cruciate ligament, the anterior motion of the lateral portion of the tibia will be more pronounced than that of the medial portion. The anterior motion of the medial portion of the tibial plateau increases relative to that of the lateral portion as the number of injured medial structures increases. Increasing anterior motion of the medial tibial plateau in turn increases the severity of the subluxation and subsequent reduction phenomenon observed by the examiner. This reduction will also be observed to occur at an increasingly high degree of flexion.

### Modified Pivot Shift Test

**Procedure:**    The patient is supine. With one hand, the examiner holds the patient's lower leg in internal rotation while the other hand grasps the tibial head laterally and holds it in a valgus position. In a positive test, this alone will produce anterior subluxation of the lateral tibial head. The rest of the procedure is identical to the pivot shift test. Subsequently flexing the knee while maintaining internal rotation and valgus stress on the lower leg causes posterior reduction of the subluxated tibial head at about 30° of flexion. The test is performed with the femoral head in abduction and adduction and in each case with the lower leg in external and internal rotation.

**Assessment:**    The iliotibial tract plays an important role in subluxation as the knee approaches extension and in subsequent reduction as flexion increases in the pivot shift test. The initial stress present in the iliotibial tract greatly influences the severity of subluxation. The iliotibial tract is relaxed in hip abduction, whereas it is under tension in hip adduction.

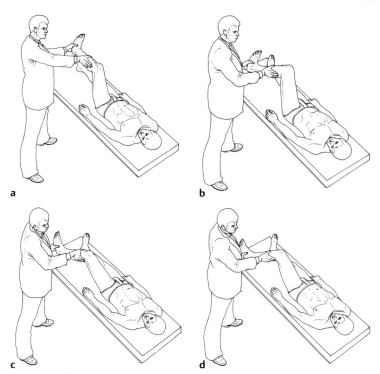

Fig. 6.**42a–d** Modified pivot shift test:
**a** subluxation during extension of the adducted leg with valgus stress and lower leg internally rotated;
**b** reduction during flexion of the leg from the same position;
**c** subluxation during extension of the abducted leg with valgus stress on the knee and lower leg externally rotated;
**d** reduction during flexion of the leg from the same position

The iliotibial tract contributes directly and indirectly (passively) to stabilizing the lateral knee. The portion of the iliotibial tract between the fibers of Kaplan and Gerdy's tubercle can be regarded as a passive ligament-like structure that is placed under tension by the proximal portion of the tract that courses through the thigh. The tension in this passive femorotibial portion of the tract determines the degree of subluxation of the tibial head. Internally rotating the lower leg and adducting the hip tenses the entire iliotibial tract, which increases tension in the ligament-like portion that spans the knee. This tension will prevent anterior subluxation of the tibial head during the pivot shift test in the presence of a torn anterior cruciate ligament. However, externally rotating the lower leg reduces the tension in the portion of the iliotibial tract that spans the knee, allowing greater anterior subluxation of the tibial head. The degree of subluxation is even greater when the leg is abducted.

### Medial Shift Test

**Procedure:**   The examiner immobilizes the patient's lower leg between his or her forearm and waist to evaluate the medial or lateral translation (tibial displacement) as the knee approaches extension. To assess medial translation, the examiner places one hand on the lower leg slightly distal to the medial joint cavity while the other hand rests on the lateral thigh. While applying a valgus stress to the knee via the lower leg, the examiner presses medially with the hand resting on the patient's thigh.

**Assessment:**   In an anterior cruciate tear, the tibia can be displaced medially until the intercondylar eminence comes in contact with the medial femoral condyle. Because the posterior cruciate ligament courses from medial to lateral, lateral translation of the tibial head will be detectable in the presence of a posterior cruciate tear (positive lateral shift test).

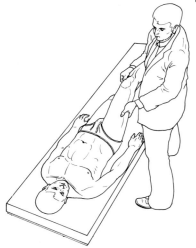

Fig. 6.**43**    Medial shift test

## Soft Pivot Shift Test

**Procedure:**  The patient is supine. The examiner grasps the patient's foot with one hand and the calf with the other. First, the examiner alternately flexes and extends the knee carefully, using these normal everyday motion sequences to alleviate the patient's anxiety and reduce reflexive muscle tension. The patient's hip is abducted, and the foot is held in neutral or external rotation.

Next, the examiner gently applies axial compression after about 3–5 flexion and extension cycles. With the hand resting on the calf, the examiner applies a mild anterior stress.

**Assessment:**  Under axial compression and mild anterior stress, slight subluxation will occur as the knee approaches extension, with reduction occurring as flexion increases. By varying the speed of the flexion and extension cycle, the axial compression, and anteriorly directed pressure, the examiner can precisely control the intensity of the subluxation and subsequent reduction. In this test, the examiner literally feels his or her way toward the subluxation and reduction.

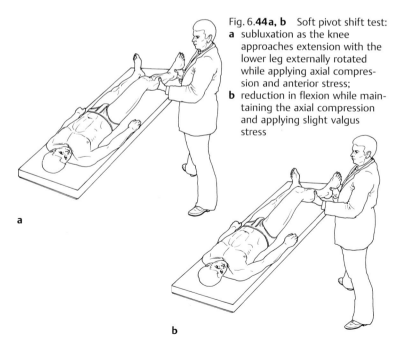

Fig. 6.**44a, b**   Soft pivot shift test:
**a** subluxation as the knee approaches extension with the lower leg externally rotated while applying axial compression and anterior stress;
**b** reduction in flexion while maintaining the axial compression and applying slight valgus stress

a

b

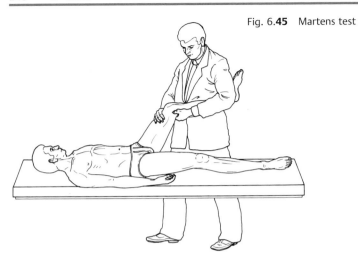

Fig. 6.**45**    Martens test

**Note:**  The soft pivot shift test ensures reduction with minimal pain or even with no pain at all. Carefully performed, this test can be repeated several times without the patient's complaining of pain.

### Martens Test

**Procedure:**  The patient is supine. The examiner stands lateral to the injured leg and immobilizes the patient's calf distal to the knee with one hand, resting the index finger on the fibula. The patient's lower leg is immobilized between the examiner's forearm and waist while a valgus stress is applied. While pulling the lower leg anteriorly with one hand, the examiner pushes the distal thigh posteriorly with the other.

**Assessment:**  The maneuver begins with the knee in a position approaching extension. As flexion is increased from this starting position, the subluxated lateral portion of the tibia will reduce at about 30° of flexion if an anterior cruciate ligament injury is present.

### Losee Test

**Procedure:**  The patient is supine. The examiner grasps the knee laterally with the thumb posterior to the fibular head and the fingers resting on the patella. The other hand grasps the lower leg medially proximal to the ankle. In contrast to the other dynamic subluxation tests, the exam-

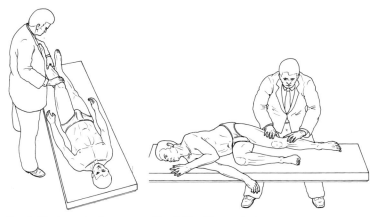

Fig. 6.**46**   Losee test          Fig. 6.**47**   Slocum test

iner does not internally rotate the lower leg but instead moves it into slight external rotation.

**Assessment:**   When the knee is extended from 40°–50° of flexion, an anterior cruciate ligament injury will lead to visible and palpable anterior subluxation of the lateral portion of the tibial head.

**Note:**   Traditionally, the external rotation of the lower leg has marked out the Losee test among the dynamic subluxation tests. However, it is important for the examiner not to force this external rotation, but to hold the lower leg in a relaxed way in external rotation with the knee flexed. Extending the knee causes the lateral portion of the tibia to subluxate anteriorly, meaning that the entire lower leg moves into internal rotation. The examiner must not interfere with this relative internal rotation.

### Slocum Test

**Procedure:**   The patient lies on the unaffected side with the hip and knee flexed, holding the injured upper leg in slight internal rotation with the foot extended where possible. In this position, the weight of the leg exerts a slight valgus stress. The examiner stands behind the patient and grasps the patient's thigh with one hand, palpating the fibular head with the thumb or index finger.

**Assessment:**   In an injury to the anterior cruciate ligament, the lateral tibial head will subluxate anteriorly with the knee in a position approaching extension. Subsequent flexion will then lead to posterior reduction of the tibial head at about 30° of flexion. This result indicates medial instability of the knee.

## Arnold Crossover Test

**Procedure:**   The examiner immobilizes the foot of the patient's injured leg. The patient then crosses the normal leg over the injured leg, rotating the pelvis and trunk toward the injured side.

**Assessment:**   The contraction of the quadriceps causes the immobilized leg to reproduce the lateral pivot shift phenomenon. The patient will experience an unpleasant sensation and report that the knee is about to dislocate.

**Note:**   In muscular patients, this test usually provides more useful diagnostic information than the other dynamic anterior cruciate ligament tests.

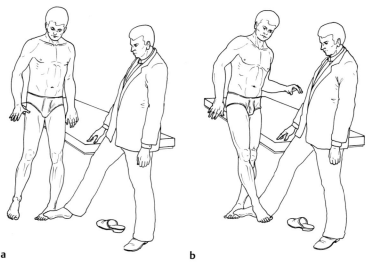

**a**                                                          **b**

Fig. 6.**48a, b**   Arnold crossover test:
**a**  starting position,
**b**  crossover

Fig. 6.**49**　Noyes test

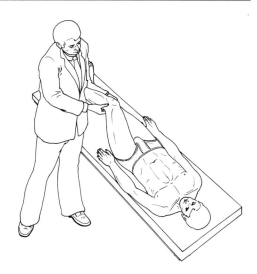

## Noyes Test

**Procedure:**　The patient is supine. The examiner grasps the tibial head with both hands and immobilizes the patient's distal lower leg between his or her forearm and waist. With the knee in about 20° of flexion, the examiner elicits a slight anterior drawer motion while simultaneously using the index fingers to evaluate whether the hamstrings are relaxed. The distal femur will drop into external rotation and slightly recede posteriorly (subluxation). The knee is then flexed from this position.

**Assessment:**　In contrast to other dynamic anterior subluxation tests, it is not the lateral portion of the tibia but the distal femur that is tested for reduction and subluxation relative to the tibial head, which the examiner immobilizes and guides posteriorly. The test is positive when knee flexion results in palpable internal rotation of the distal femur (reduction). This indicates cruciate ligament insufficiency.

**Note:**　The Noyes test is suitable for assessing cruciate ligament insufficiency in an apprehensive patient who has difficulty relaxing the hamstrings.

## Jakob Giving Way Test

**Procedure:**  The patient leans against the wall on the normal side and distributes his or her body weight over both legs. The examiner places one hand each proximal and distal to the injured knee and applies a valgus stress while the patient flexes the knee.

**Assessment:**  The test is positive when anterior subluxation of the tibial head occurs and the patient reports a subjective sensation of the knee "giving way."

## Lemaire Test

**Procedure:**  The patient is supine. The examiner internally rotates the patient's foot with one hand while pressing against the lateral thigh with the other hand, which rests proximal to the lateral femoral condyle. The examiner then carefully extends and flexes the knee.

**Assessment:**  In an anterior cruciate ligament tear, the examiner will observe anterior subluxation of the lateral tibial head as the knee approaches extension. Spontaneous reduction will then occur at 30°–50° of flexion.

**Note:**  This test method was described first by Lemaire and subsequently by Galway and McIntosh; it is often referred to by the latter names.

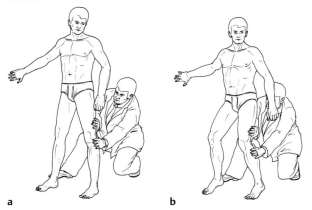

**a**                                    **b**

Fig. 6.**50a, b**   Jakob giving way test:
**a** starting position with valgus stress,
**b** reduction in flexion while maintaining valgus stress

Fig. 6.**51** Lemaire test

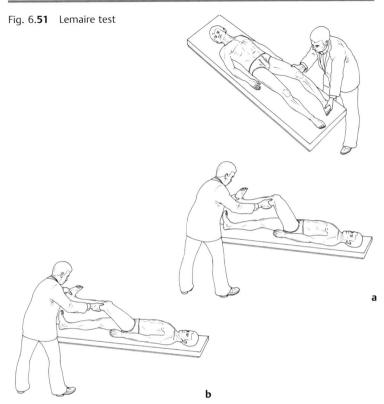

**a**

**b**

Fig. 6.**52a, b** Hughston jerk test:
**a** starting position with knee flexed 70°, lower leg internally rotated, and valgus stress applied;
**b** anterior subluxation of the lateral tibial head at 20° of flexion with the lower leg internally rotated and valgus stress applied

## Hughston Jerk Test

**Procedure:** The patient is supine with the knee flexed 60°–70°. The examiner grasps the patient's foot with one hand and internally rotates the lower leg while applying a valgus stress with the other hand.

**Assessment:** The flexed knee is extended with the tibia in slight internal rotation. In an anterior cruciate ligament tear, the lateral portion of the tibial head will abruptly subluxate anteriorly at about 20° of flexion.

**Note:**  A positive jerk test indicates that the same structures are injured as indicated by a positive pivot shift maneuver and assesses antero-lateral rotatory instability. This test is not as sensitive as the pivot shift test.

## ■ Function Tests to Assess the Posterior Cruciate Ligament

### Posterior Drawer Test in 90° Flexion (Posterior Lachman Test)

**Procedure:**  The posterior drawer test is performed with the knee in flexion and in a position approaching extension. It is similar to the anterior drawer test except that it is used to evaluate posterior translation in neutral, internal, and external rotation.

**Assessment:**  Isolated posterolateral instability exhibits maximum posterior translation with the knee in a position approaching extension. Maximum posterolateral rotation and minimum posterior drawer are observed with the knee in 90° of flexion. In an isolated posterior cruciate ligament injury, maximum posterior translation occurs in flexion, and

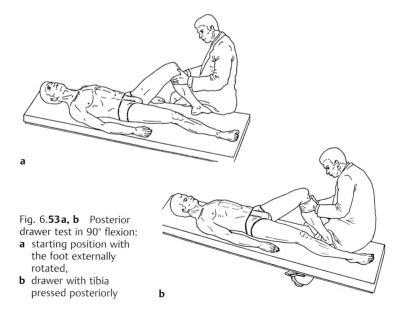

Fig. 6.**53a, b**  Posterior drawer test in 90° flexion:
**a** starting position with the foot externally rotated,
**b** drawer with tibia pressed posteriorly

posterolateral translation will be observed neither in flexion nor with the knee in a position approaching extension.

Where there is combined insufficiency of the posterior cruciate ligament and the posterolateral structures, an increased posterior drawer, external rotation, and lateral opening will be observed in all degrees of flexion.

### Reversed Jakob Pivot Shift Test

Assesses posterolateral rotational instability.

**Procedure:** The patient is supine. The examiner stands on the side of injured leg. With one hand, the examiner grasps the patient's foot while the other hand supports the lateral aspect of the lower leg at the level of the knee. The thumb of this hand palpates the fibular head and applies valgus pressure. The examiner now flexes the patient's knee 70°–80°. Externally rotating the foot in this position causes posterior subluxation of the lateral tibial plateau. The examiner then slowly extends the knee while maintaining slight valgus stress.

**Assessment:** In the presence of a posterolateral injury with the knee flexed, the tibia follows gravity and drops into posterolateral subluxation. Externally rotating the tibia increases this subluxation. As the knee is then extended and passes through 30°–20° of flexion, the iliotibial tract begins to act as an extensor and reduces the joint. The posterolateral capsule, the posterior soft tissue envelope of the knee, and the quadriceps also contribute to the reduction.

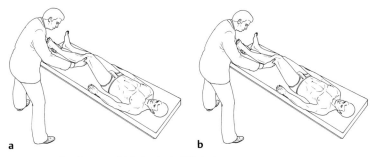

Fig. 6.**54a, b**   Reversed Jakob pivot shift test:
**a** posterior subluxation of the tibia with knee flexed more than 60°,
**b** reduction as the knee approaches extension

**Note:** This test is the functional counterpart of the dynamic anterior subluxation test. However, it can be positive in patients with increased generalized laxity of the ligaments. This test is only clinically significant when a positive result can be elicited unilaterally and faithfully reproduces the painful subluxation symptoms described by the patient. A positive test primarily suggests a posterolateral capsular ligament injury. Injury to the posterior cruciate ligament is likely in patients with a history of trauma and simultaneous posterolateral instability in the form of a positive posterior drawer when the lower leg is in external rotation.

### Quadriceps Contraction Test

Assesses a posterior cruciate ligament injury.

**Procedure:** The patient is supine. The injured leg is flexed 90° at the knee and placed in external rotation. The patient is asked tense the quadriceps and lift the leg off the examining table.

**Assessment:** In the presence of posterolateral instability, the external rotation of the foot causes posterior subluxation of the lateral tibia relative to the lateral femoral condyle. The examiner observes this as a posterior droop of the lateral tibial plateau. The active quadriceps contraction and increasing knee extension cause the lateral tibial plateau to move anteriorly out of posterior subluxation and into reduction with a sort of reverse pivot shift. The joint reduces at about 30°–20° of flexion. This test is also called an active reduction test and can usually be demonstrated only in the presence of chronic ligament injuries.

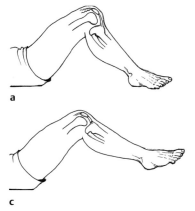

a

b

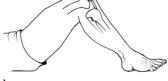

Fig. 6.**55a–c**   Quadriceps contraction test:
**a** subluxation with posterior droop,
**b** tensing the quadriceps,
**c** active knee extension: reduction position

c

## Posterior Drop Test

**Procedure:**   Both knees are held parallel in 90° of flexion.

**Assessment:**   Inspecting the silhouettes of both tibial heads from the side reveals that the tibial head in the affected knee appears to "droop." The rest position of the posterior drawer is influenced by gravity and is a sensitive sign of a posterior cruciate ligament injury.

## Soft Posterolateral Drawer Test

**Procedure:**   The patient is seated with the legs relaxed and hanging over the edge of the table. The foot of the affected leg rests lightly on the thigh of the examiner, who crouches in front of the patient. The examiner grasps the tibial head with both hands and presses it posteriorly with the balls of the thumbs.

**Assessment:**   Posterior translation (drawer motion) of the lateral tibial plateau is a sign of posterolateral instability.

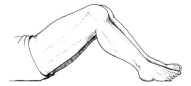

Fig. 6.**56**   Posterior drop test

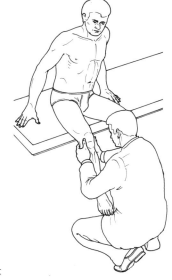

Fig. 6.**57**   Soft posterolateral drawer test

## Gravity Sign and Genu Recurvatum Test

**Procedure:**   The patient is supine with the hip and knee of the affected leg flexed 90°. With one hand, the examiner grasps the patient's lower leg while stabilizing the knee proximal to the patella with the other hand. The examiner then abruptly pulls away the stabilizing hand from the knee.

**Assessment:**   If the posterior cruciate ligament is torn, the tibia will recede posteriorly (posterior droop).

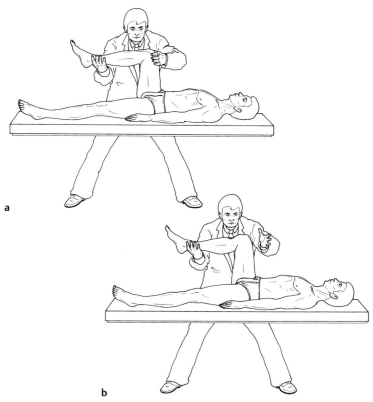

Fig. 6.**58a, b**   Gravity sign and genu recurvatum test:
**a** stabilizing the joint,
**b** posterior droop of the tibia after removal of stabilization

**Note:** In the genu recurvatum test, the extended leg is lifted. A torn posterior cruciate ligament will result in a posterior droop of the tibia.

## Hughston Test for Genu Recurvatum and External Rotation

**Procedure:** The patient is supine with both quadriceps completely relaxed. The examiner then lifts each forefoot.

**Assessment:** In posterolateral instability, this maneuver will produce a hyperextended varus position in the knee with simultaneous external rotation of the tibia.

**Note:** To demonstrate the external rotation and genu recurvatum deformity (hyperextension) more clearly, the test may be performed on one leg at a time. This is done by moving the knee from slight flexion into extension. The examiner places one hand on the posterior aspect of the knee to palpate the posterior droop and the slight external rotation of the proximal tibia.

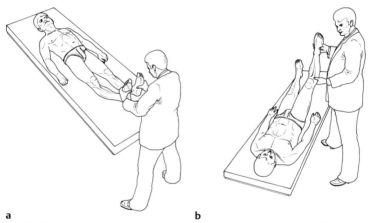

**a**                              **b**

Fig. 6.**59a, b**   Hughston test for genu recurvatum and external rotation:
**a** hyperextended varus position,
**b** flexion into extension movement

## Godfrey Test

**Procedure:**  The patient is supine with both knees and hips flexed 90°. The examiner holds the patient's lower legs while pressing the tibial tuberosity of the injured knee posteriorly.

**Assessment:**  Even in the starting position, the examiner will readily notice the slight posterior droop in the proximal tibia indicative of posterior cruciate ligament insufficiency. Applying pressure to the anterior tibia increases the posterior droop of the lateral tibial plateau.

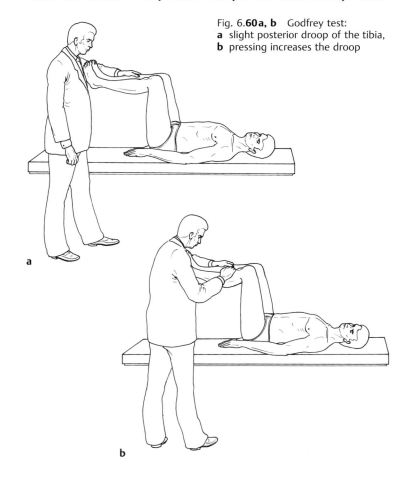

Fig. 6.**60a, b**   Godfrey test:
**a**  slight posterior droop of the tibia,
**b**  pressing increases the droop

a

b

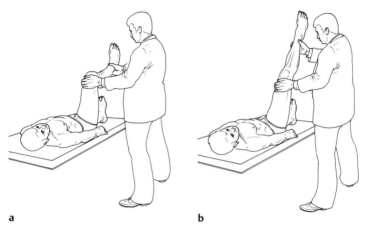

**a**          **b**
Fig. 6.**61 a, b**   Dynamic posterior shift test:
**a** subluxation with hip and knee flexed 90°,
**b** reduction as the knee approaches extension

## Dynamic Posterior Shift Test

**Procedure:** The patient is supine. The examiner passively flexes the hip and knee of the affected leg 90°, holding the knee in neutral rotation. One of the examiner's hands rests on the thigh and acts as a buttress while the examiner slowly extends the knee with the other hand.

**Assessment:** Once the knee reaches about 20° of flexion, the examiner will be able to observe and palpate an abrupt movement of the tibial plateau out of posterior subluxation into reduction and external rotation.

## Loomer Posterolateral Rotary Instability Test

**Procedure:** The patient lies supine and flexes both hips and both knees to 90°. The examiner then grasps the feet and maximally laterally rotates both tibias.

**Assessment:** The test is considered positive if the injured tibia laterally rotates excessively and there is posterior sag of the effected tibial tubercle; both signs must be present for a positive test. Other authors describe a modification of the Loomer test which is called the tibial external rotation test or Dial test.

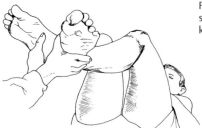

Fig. 6.**62**   Loomer posterolateral instability test: flexion of the hips and knees to 90°

The patient may be placed in the supine or prone position. The examiner flexes the knee to 30°, extends the foot over the side of the examining table and stabilizes the femur on the table. The examiner then laterally rotates the tibia on the femur and compares the amount of rotation to that on the good side.

If the test is performed with the patient supine, the examiner can observe and compare the amount of tibial tubercle movement . The test is then repeated with the knee flexed to 90° and the thigh still on the examining table. If the tibia rotates less at 90° than at 30°, an isolated posterolateral (popliteus corner) injury is more likely. If the knee rotates more at 90°, injury to both the popliteus corner and posterior cruciate are more likely.

# 7 Lower Leg, Ankle, and Foot

Lesions of the ankle and foot can alter the mechanics of gait and as a result cause stress on other lower limb joints. The foot and ankle combine flexibility with stability because of the many bones, their shapes, and their attachments. The lower leg, ankle, and foot have two principle functions: propulsion and support. For propulsion they act like a flexible lever. For support they act like a rigid structure that holds up the entire body. When assessing the lower leg, ankle, and foot it is important to always assess the neutral position of the foot in both weight-bearing and nonweight-bearing situations. This will help the examiner to differentiate functional from structural deformities.

Age, gender, occupation, and leisure activities are factors to consider in every patient. It is important to enquire about the character of the onset of pain, its location and radiation, its nature, and about factors that can cause pain. Both feet and the adjacent joints such as the knee should be examined and assessed comparatively. Axial deviations in the legs should also be given consideration. Inspection of the shape and soles of the patient's shoes is important as asymmetric wear on the soles may provide an initial indication of the cause of the patient's complaints.

In addition to a palpatory examination with assessment of mobility and tenderness to palpation in the specific region, it is important to observe the foot during weight bearing and walking. Metatarsalgia is a general term for pain in the forefoot. Splay foot is the most common deformity of the foot and the most common cause of metatarsalgia. The collapse of the transverse metatarsal arch as a result of weakness of the muscles and ligaments leads to secondary changes in the foot with claw toe and hammer toe deformities and hallux valgus. Plantar calluses from the increased stresses on the metatarsal heads in turn lead to additional problems. Other causes of forefoot pain include osteoarthritis (hallux rigidus), neuromas (Morton neuroma), stress fractures, avascular necrosis (Koehler disease), disorders of the sesamoids, plantar warts, and compression neuropathies (tarsal tunnel syndrome).

Certain systemic diseases tend to involve the foot. Often the first clinical symptoms of these disorders will appear in the foot. Such disorders include diabetes mellitus, peripheral arterial disease, gout, psoriasis, collagen disorders, and rheumatoid arthritis.

## ■ Range of Motion in the Ankle and Foot (Neutral-Zero Method)

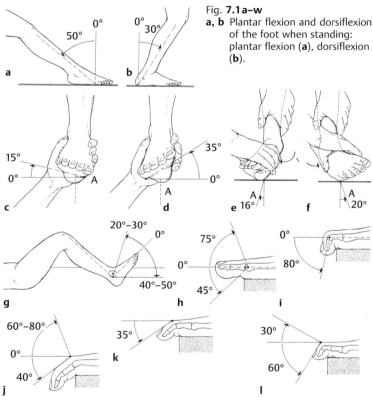

Fig. **7.1a–w**

**a, b** Plantar flexion and dorsiflexion of the foot when standing: plantar flexion (**a**), dorsiflexion (**b**).

**c, d** Pronation (**c**) and supination (**d**) of the forefoot. One hand grasps the heel and the other turns the forefoot. Only the angle of the forefoot relative to the hindfoot is measured as pronation and supination.

**e, f** Eversion (**e**) and inversion (**f**) of the hindfoot. One hand grasps the lower leg and the other grasps the posterior aspect of the forefoot, holding the calcaneus between thumb and forefinger (not shown). The inversion and eversion is evaluated on the calcaneus (axis of the calcaneus, A). Care should be taken to avoid pronation or supination of the foot.

**g** Plantar flexion and dorsiflexion of the ankle (talocrural joint) with the foot hanging relaxed.

**h–l** Motion in the metatarsophalangeal joints: great toe (**h, i**), other toes (**j–l**).

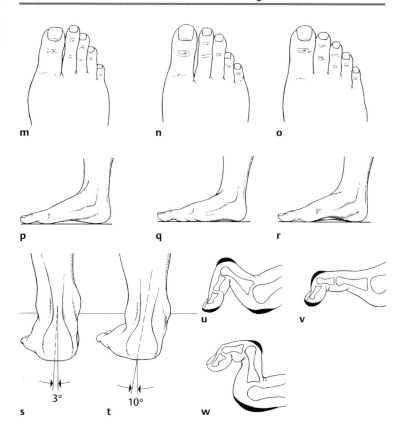

Fig. **7.1**

**m–o**  The most common variations in forefoot and toe length: Greek (**m**), square (**n**), and Egyptian as described by Lelièvre (**o**).

**p–r**  Assessment of the medial longitudinal arch of the foot: normal arch rising slightly above the floor (**p**), absent arch or flatfoot (**q**), abnormally high arch or pes cavus (**r**).

**s, t**  Assessment of the position of the hindfoot. Normal position is a valgus angle of 0°–6°. A valgus angle exceeding 6° is pes valgus; any varus angle is pes varus.

**u–w**  The most important toe deformities: hammer toe in the proximal interphalangeal joint (**u**), hammer toe in the distal interphalangeal joint (**v**), claw toe as described by Lelièvre (**w**).

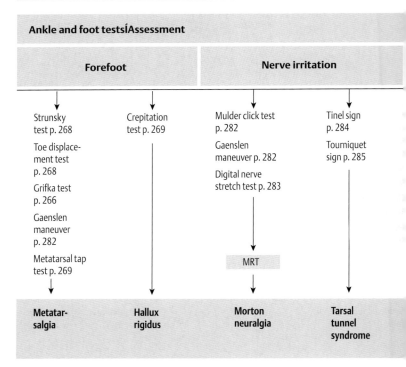

Fig. 7.**2**   Ankle and foot tests

## ■ Function Tests

### Grifka Test

Assesses splay foot.

**Procedure:**   After passively dorsiflexing the toes of one foot, the examiner applies distal and plantar finger pressure to longitudinally compress the metatarsal heads in the metatarsophalangeal joints.

**Assessment:**   This compression corresponds to the transfer of compressive forces to the metatarsal heads in the painful toe-off phase of walking. With a splay foot, this is often painful while plantar compression alone is painless.

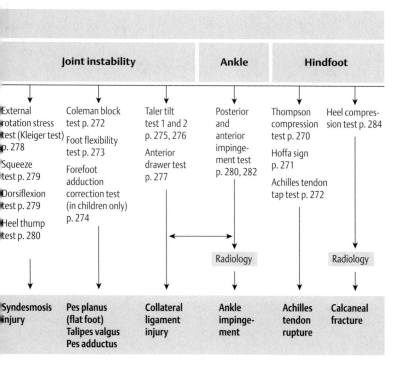

| | Joint instability | | Ankle | Hindfoot | |
|---|---|---|---|---|---|
| **External rotation stress test (Kleiger test) p. 278** | Coleman block test p. 272 | Taler tilt test 1 and 2 p. 275, 276 | Posterior and anterior impingement test p. 280, 282 | Thompson compression test p. 270 | Heel compression test p. 284 |
| **Squeeze test p. 279** | Foot flexibility test p. 273 | Anterior drawer test p. 277 | | Hoffa sign p. 271 | |
| **Dorsiflexion test p. 279** | Forefoot adduction correction test (in children only) p. 274 | | | Achilles tendon tap test p. 272 | |
| **Heel thump test p. 280** | | | | | |
| | | | Radiology | | Radiology |
| ↓ | ↓ | ↓ | ↓ | ↓ | ↓ |
| **Syndesmosis injury** | **Pes planus (flat foot) Talipes valgus Pes adductus** | **Collateral ligament injury** | **Ankle impinge-ment** | **Achilles tendon rupture** | **Calcaneal fracture** |

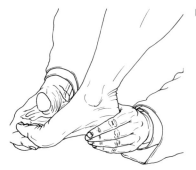

Fig. 7.**3** Grifka test

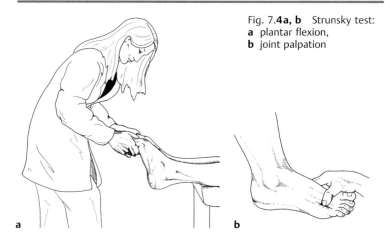

Fig. 7.**4a, b**   Strunsky test:
**a** plantar flexion,
**b** joint palpation

a                                                                    b

### Strunsky Test

Provocation test to assess metatarsalgia.

**Procedure:**   The patient is supine with the feet hanging over the edge of the examining table. With each great toe between the thumb and index finger, the examiner grasps the patient's other toes in a pincer grip and forcefully plantar flexes the metatarsophalangeal joints.

**Assessment:**   Where there is chronic irritation of the metatarsophalangeal joints with metatarsalgia, this test significantly increases symptoms as a result of the increased pressure on the metatarsophalangeal joints. Subsequent palpation of the metatarsophalangeal joints can then identify the painful joint.

### Toe Displacement Test

Tests instability of the metatarsophalangeal joints.

**Procedure:**   While immobilizing the medial forefoot with one hand, the examiner grasps the distal portion of one proximal phalanx with the other hand and moves it posteriorly and plantarward relative to the metatarsal head.

**Assessment:**   Motion pain in the metatarsophalangeal joint accompanied by signs of instability suggests an increasing deformity of the toe leading to a functional claw toe deformity during weight bearing. Pro-

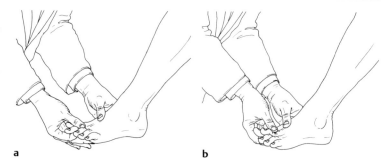

Fig. 7.**5**   Toe displacement test:
**a** posterior displacement,
**b** plantar displacement

gression of this instability leads to a permanent claw toe deformity with the metatarsophalangeal joint fixed in dorsiflexion.

In a dislocation of the metatarsophalangeal joint, it will be impossible to reduce the joint in the toe displacement test. The result is metatarsalgia with development of plantar calluses.

## Crepitation Test

Indicates hallux rigidus.

**Procedure:**  With the patient's foot relaxed and hanging, the examiner approaches from distally and grasps the proximal phalanx of the great toe, with his or her thumb on its posterior aspect and fingers on its plantar aspect. The examiner immobilizes the lateral forefoot with the other hand, placing the thumb on its plantar aspect and the fingers on its posterior aspect. The examiner passively plantar flexes, dorsiflexes, and rotates the metatarsophalangeal joint.

**Assessment:**  In hallux rigidus, joint motion in every direction will be painful and, primarily in dorsiflexion, restricted. This will be accompanied by palpable or audible crepitation as a result of osteoarthritic changes in the joint.

## Metatarsal Tap Test

Provocation test for assessment of metatarsalgia.

**Procedure:**  The patient is supine with the feet hanging over the edge of the examining table. The examiner slightly hyperextends the toes with

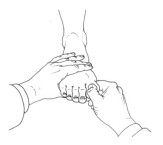

Fig. 7.**6**   Crepitation test

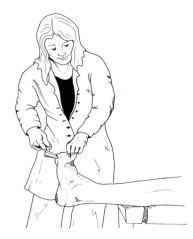

Fig. 7.**7**   Metatarsal tap test

one hand and taps the metatarsal heads or metatarsophalangeal joints with a reflex hammer held in the other hand.

**Assessment:**   In a patient with metatarsalgia due to chronic irritation of the metatarsophalangeal joints, tapping the ball of the foot will exacerbate the metatarsalgia symptoms. Pain upon tapping that occurs between the metatarsal heads—primarily the third and fourth metatarsals—with acute episodic pain radiating into the adjacent toes suggests a Morton neuroma (see Mulder click test).

### Thompson Compression Test (Calf Compression Test)

Indicates an Achilles tendon tear.

**Procedure:**   The patient is prone with the feet projecting past the edge of the examining table. The examiner grasps the calf of the affected leg with one hand and forcefully compresses the musculature.

**Assessment:**   Compressing the calf muscles should normally provoke rapid passive plantar flexion of the foot. Absence of this plantar flexion suggests a torn Achilles tendon. The response to the compression test is not always unambiguous in patients with partial tears and will depend on the degree of disruption. In an Achilles tendon tear, the patient will be unable to stand on tiptoe, especially when standing only on the injured leg, and the Achilles tendon reflex will be absent.

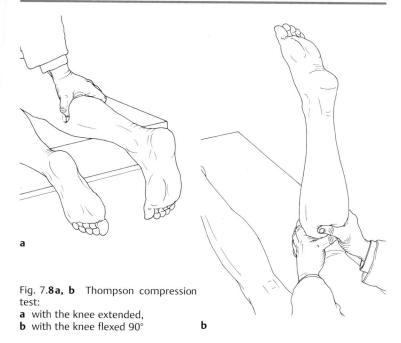

Fig. 7.**8a, b** Thompson compression test:
**a** with the knee extended,
**b** with the knee flexed 90°

**Note:** The test can also be performed with the patient prone and the knee flexed 90°. In this position, the examiner grasps the patient's calf with both hands and forcefully compresses the musculature. Loss of plantar flexion is a sign of an Achilles tendon tear (Simmond test).

### Hoffa Sign

Indicates a chronic Achilles tendon tear.

**Procedure:** The patient is prone with the feet projecting over the edge of the examining table. The examiner passively dorsiflexes both feet.

**Assessment:** In a chronic Achilles tendon tear, tension in the Achilles tendon will be reduced and the affected foot can be dorsiflexed farther than the contralateral foot. The patient is then requested to stand on tiptoe on each leg. This will be impossible with an Achilles tendon tear in the injured leg.

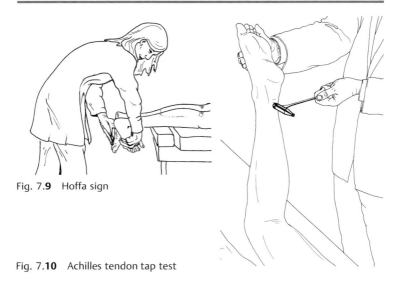

Fig. 7.**9**   Hoffa sign

Fig. 7.**10**   Achilles tendon tap test

## Achilles Tendon Tap Test

Indicates an Achilles tendon tear.

**Procedure:**   The patient is prone with the knee flexed 90°. The examiner taps the distal third of the Achilles tendon with a reflex hammer.

**Assessment:**   Increased pain and loss of plantar flexion (Achilles tendon reflex) are signs of a tear in the Achilles tendon. In the absence of an Achilles tendon reflex, a differential diagnosis should exclude neurologic changes.

## Coleman Block Test

Flexibility test for assessment of hindfoot deformities.

**Procedure:**   The patient is standing. The lateral block test involves placing wooden blocks of varying height beneath the heel and the lateral margin of the foot. The blocks are placed according to the severity and shape of the foot deformity so as to allow the first metatarsal to reach the floor. In the medial block test, the wooden block must be placed beneath the first metatarsal head.

**Assessment:**   The block test is a good method for determining the flexibility of compensatory hindfoot deformities in the presence of

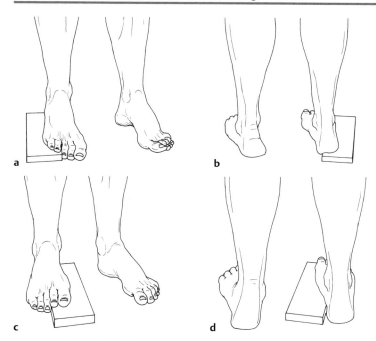

Fig. 7.**11a–d**   Coleman block test:
**a** hindfoot varus and forefoot valgus viewed from the front,
**b** hindfoot varus and forefoot valgus viewed from the rear,
**c** hindfoot valgus and forefoot varus viewed from the front,
**d** hindfoot valgus and forefoot varus viewed from the rear

simultaneous fixed forefoot contractures. The lateral block test is used to determine the flexibility of a varus hindfoot deformity in the presence of a simultaneous valgus forefoot contracture. A flexible compensatory varus hindfoot deformity will be corrected by the lateral block. Where a varus forefoot contracture is present, the medial block test will allow evaluation of the flexibility and/or severity of the contracture in the hindfoot deformity.

## Foot Flexibility Test

Assesses rigid or flexible talipes planovalgus deformity.

**Procedure:**   Talipes planovalgus is a foot deformity in which the medial longitudinal arch of the foot is flattened (flatfoot, talipes planus, or pes

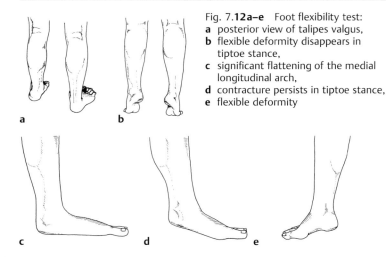

Fig. 7.**12a–e**   Foot flexibility test:
**a**  posterior view of talipes valgus,
**b**  flexible deformity disappears in
      tiptoe stance,
**c**  significant flattening of the medial
      longitudinal arch,
**d**  contracture persists in tiptoe stance,
**e**  flexible deformity

planus) and the valgus position of the heel is increased (talipes valgus). The feet are examined from the side and from behind with the patient standing in the normal position and on tiptoe.

**Assessment:**   Persistent flattening of the medial longitudinal arch and persistent valgus position of the heel when the patient stands on tiptoe indicate a rigid talipes planovalgus deformity. In a flexible talipes planovalgus deformity, the tiptoe stance will bring about a varus shift in the heel to compensate for the valgus deformity, and the medial longitudinal arch will reappear.

## Forefoot Adduction Correction Test

For assessment and differential diagnosis of rigid and flexible pes adductus.

**Procedure:**   The child is supine. The examiner grasps the foot of the affected leg with one hand and attempts to correct the pes adductus deformity by pressing on the medial aspect of the forefoot with thumb of the other hand.

**Assessment:**   Where this maneuver readily moves the forefoot across the midline and eliminates the pes adductus, the deformity is usually flexible and will be spontaneously corrected. A deformity that cannot be passively corrected is a rigid pes adductus.

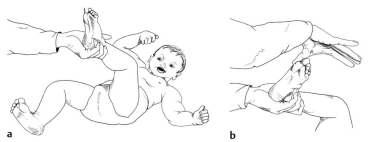

Fig. 7.**13a, b**   Forefoot adduction correction test:
**a** deformity,
**b** passively correctable

Congenital pes adductus deformities that resist manual correction will require rigorous timely treatment in corrective plaster casts.

## Collateral and Syndesmosis Ligaments

The distal syndesmotic articulation between the tibia and fibula is comprised of three major ligaments: the anterior inferior tibiofibular ligament, the posterior inferior tibiofibular ligament, and the interosseous ligament.

These ligaments provide such strong stabilization to the articulation that the fibula only rotates externally up to 2° relative to the tibia and the ankle mortise widens only about 1 mm as the intact ankle joint moves from full plantar flexion to full dorsiflexion.

The mechanisms for syndesmotic injury include external rotation of the foot, eversion of the talus within the ankle mortise, and excessive dorsiflexion.

The mechanism of injury for the deltoid ligament is similar to syndesmotic injuries, involving external rotation of the foot or eversion of the talus within the ankle mortise.

The mechanism of collateral ligament ruptures involves a supination-inversion motion with the foot in slight plantar flexion. The anterior talofibular ligament and the calcaneofibular ligament tear sequentially; the posterior talofibular ligament (the strongest ligament) is rarely injured.

## Talar Tilt Test 1 (Inversion Stress Test or Varus Stress Test)

Testing the integrity of the calcaneofibular and anterior talofibular ligament.

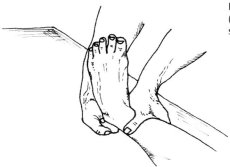

Fig. 7.**14**   Talar tilt test 1 (inversion stress test or varus stress test)

**Procedure:**   The patient is lying supine or sitting with legs over the edge of the examination table. The examiner holds the calcaneus with one hand in order to bring the foot and ankle into the neutral position. The other hand stabilizes the lower leg. The thumb or the fingers are placed along the calcaneofibular ligament, so that any gapping of the talus away from the mortise can be felt. The hand holding the calcaneus applies inverse stress by pushing the calcaneus medially and by this causing the talus to tilt.

**Assessment:**   Obvious strong angulation or a difference of more than 15° between both ankles is suggestive of complete tears of both the calcaneofibular and anterior talofibular ligament on the unaffected side. Maximum dorsal flexion locking the subtalar joint may improve the sensitivity of this test. However, it is important to examine both ankles, because in some individuals (especially children) lax joints are more common and physiologic.

This test may be best appreciated when test outcomes are interpreted together with the drawer test results. Comparing the findings of both tests can be useful for differentiating isolated anterior abnormalities of the talofibulare ligament and bilateral ligament abnormalities (of the anterior talofibular and calcaneofibular ligament).

### Talar Tilt Test 2 (Eversion Stress Test or Valgus Stress Test)

Testing for the integrity of the deltoid ligament, especially the tibiocalcanea ligament.

**Procedure:**   The patient is lying or sitting with both legs hanging from the edge of the examination table. One hand grasps the calcaneus and keeps the foot in a neutral position. The other hand stabilizes the lower

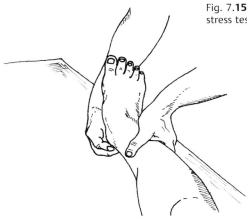

Fig. 7.**15** Talar tilt test 2 (eversion stress test or valgus stress test)

leg and the thumb or fingers are placed along the deltoid ligament. In this way, any gapping between the talus and mortise can be felt.

The hand holding the calcaneus pushes it laterally, tilting the talus and causing a gap to open on the medial side of the ankle mortise.

**Assessment:** An injury of the deltoid ligament is likely when the talus tilts or gaps excessively in comparison to the uninjured side or if pain is described during the test.

### Anterior Drawer Test

Testing for the integrity of the anterior talofibular ligament.

**Procedure:** The knee joint of the supine patient must be kept in flexion (30°) to neutralize the pull of the gastrocnemius. The ankle joint has to be fixed in 10°–15° plantar flexion and the heel is grasped with one hand. The patient's foot lies on the anterior aspect of the examiner's forearm. With the other hand the examiner holds back the tibia. Before performing the test, the patient has to relax his muscles. The heel is then very gently pressed forward, while applying a stabilizing force to the tibia.

**Assessment:** In the presence of a rupture of the anterior talofibular ligament (and the associated capsule) the talus (and thus the foot) rotates anteriorly under the ankle mortise. The center of rotation is the intact ligament. The test indicates anterior talofibular ligament instability, which is usually secondary to rupture.

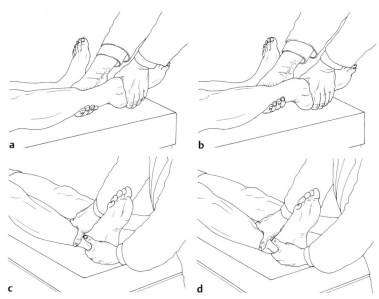

Fig. 7.**16a–d**   Drawer test:
**a** starting position,
**b** foot is pushed,
**c** starting position,
**d** foot is pulled anteriorly

## External Rotation Stress Test (Kleiger Test)

**Procedure:**   The patient is sitting at the edge of the examination table. The examiner stabilizes the proximal leg with one hand, while the other hand applies an external rotation load to the foot with the ankle positioned in neutral dorsiflexion/plantar flexion.

**Assessment:**   The external rotation load imposed on the foot rotates the talus externally and promotes lateral displacement of the fibula and increased separation of the distal syndesmosis.

Pain experienced at the anterolateral aspect of the distal tibiofibular syndesmosis is a positive sign for syndesmosis injury.

Pain on the medial side of the injured ankle during the external rotation stress test, with the ankle positioned in plantar flexion, may indicate involvement of the deltoid ligament.

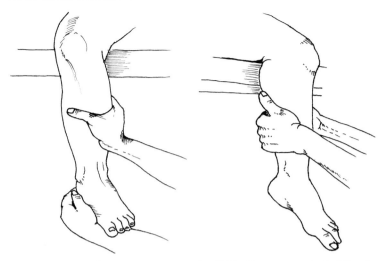

Fig. 7.**17**   External rotation stress test
(Kleiger test): test for syndesmosis injury

Fig. 7.**18**   Squeeze test: test of the distal syndesmosis ligament

## Squeeze Test

**Procedure:**  The patient sits at the edge of the examination table. The
examiner cups both hands around the distal fibula und tibia and compresses the leg, followed by application of the same load at successively
more proximal locations until pain is noticed at the distal tibiofibular
syndesmosis. The purpose of the sequentially more proximal squeezing
is to avoid unexpected and intense pain at the injured syndesmosis.

**Assessment:**  The presence of pain at the distal tibiofibular syndesmosis indicates disruption of the distal syndesmosis ligaments.

## Dorsiflexion Test

**Procedure:**  The patient sits at the edge of the examination table and
the examiner stabilizes the patient's leg with one hand, while the
examiners other hand passively moves the foot into dorsiflexion.

**Assessment:**  Pain experienced at the distal tibiofibular syndesmosis is
a positive test result.

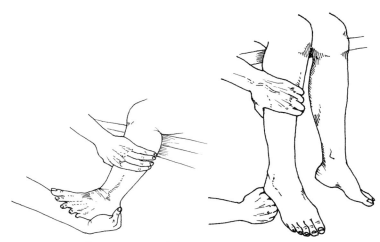

Fig. 7.**19**  Dorsiflexion test: test of tibio-fibular syndesmosis

Fig. 7.**20**  Heel thump test: test of tibiofibular syndesmosis injury

### Heel Thump Test

**Procedure:**  The patient sits at the edge of the examination table with the ankle resting in plantar flexion. The examiner holds the patient's leg with one hand and with the other hand applies a gentle but firm thump on the heel with their fist. This force is applied at the center of the heel and in line with the long axis of the tibia.

**Assessment:**  Pain experienced at the distal tibiofibular syndesmosis suggests the presence of injury.

Although the heel thump test has been recommended to help differentiate between a syndesmotic sprain and a lateral ankle sprain, this test may not be specific for a syndesmotic sprain, because this test has also been recommended to assess the possible presence of tibial stress fractures.

### Posterior Ankle Impingement Test—Hyperplantar Flexion Test

**Procedure:**  With one hand the examiner holds the patient's heel and stabilizes the back of mid- and forefoot with the other. The sitting patient's legs hang over the edge of the table and the knees are in 90°

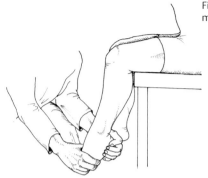

Fig. 7.**21**   Posterior ankle impingement test—hyperplantar flexion test

of flexion. The examiner then forces the foot into maximum plantar-
flexion.

The test should be performed as a series of repetitive quick passive
movements as described above.

It can be repeated in slight external or internal rotation of the foot in
relation to the tibia.

**Assessment:**   A bony or soft tissue impediment will become impacted
between the tibia and the calcaneus leading to sharp pain.

With the foot in maximum plantar flexion the examiner can also
apply a rotating force to the foot. This cause the posterior talar process
and/or os trigonum to grind between the tibia and calcaneus.

A negative test rules out a posterior impingement syndrome.

A positive test combined with pain felt on posterolateral palpation
should be followed by a diagnostic infiltration.

The capsule should be infiltrated on the posterolateral aspect of the
foot between the prominent talar process and the posterior edge of the
tibia. For example Xylocain can be used as local anaesthetic. If, in forced
plantar flexion, the pain disappears, the diagnosis is confirmed.

**Note:**   The posterior ankle impingement syndrome due to overuse is
most commonly seen in ballet dancers and runners. Downhill running
can impose repetitive stresses to the posterior aspect of the ankle joint.
The "en pointe" or the "demi-pointe" position is achieved by forceful
plantar flexion which results in compression of the posterior aspect of
the ankle joint. Therefore, posterolateral foot pain in dancers is also
called "dancers heel."

Structural abnormalities like a displaced os trigonum, a hypertrophic
posterior talar process, a thickened posterior capsule, posttraumatic

scar tissue or calcifications, loose bodies located in the posterior part of the ankle joint or osteophytes at the distal end of tibia may cause symptoms due to compression caused by excessive plantar flexion.

## Anterior Ankle Impingement Test—Hyperdorsiflexion Test

Local pain felt on palpation of the anterior joint line is most commonly located medially or laterally to the tibialis anterior muscle and the extensor digitorum longus muscle. Tibial osteophytes, osteophytes at the talar neck and soft tissue inflammation can be the reason for the anterior ankle impingement syndrome.

Forced hyperdorsiflexion may provoke this pain. However, false negative results are common.

## Gaenslen Maneuver

Assessment of forefoot pain.

**Procedure:**   The examiner immobilizes the metatarsal heads in one plane between the fingers of one hand on the plantar aspect of the foot and the thumb on the posterior aspect. The other hand grasps the toes in a pincer grip, applying medial and lateral compression to the forefoot via the metatarsal heads of the great toe and little toe.

**Assessment:**   This forefoot "pincer grip" will elicit pain between the metatarsal heads, often with acute episodic pain radiating into the adjacent toes, in the presence of a Morton neuroma (a painful interdigital neuroma). It will also often cause pain in a significant splay foot deformity where there is irritation of the joint capsule.

## Mulder Click Test (Morton Test)

Indicates an interdigital neuroma (Morton neuroma).

**Procedure:**   The examiner grasps the patient's forefoot in a pincer grip and presses it together. This pushes the adjacent metatarsal heads against each other.

**Assessment:**   Where an interdigital neuroma is present, pushing the metatarsal heads against one another will cause pain with occasional paresthesia radiating into the adjacent toes. Small fibroma-like hardened areas between the toes will also be palpable and will displace, sometimes with a clicking sound, as the forefoot is compressed. Morton neuroma is a spindle-shaped bulb that develops in a plantar nerve. Painful interdigital neuromas usually develop in the second or third

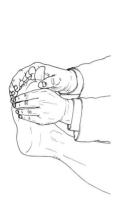

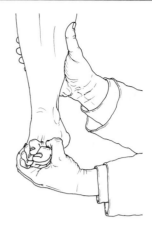

Fig. 7.**22**   Gaenslen maneuver      Fig. 7.**23**   Mulder click test

interdigital fold; neuromas in the first or fourth interdigital fold are rare. Injection of a local anesthetic through the deep transverse metatarsal ligament can confirm the diagnosis by anesthetizing the neuroma. Pressure also indicates metatarsalgia.

## Digital Nerve Stretch Test

**Procedure:**   The patient lies supine. Both ankles are held in full dorsiflexion, while the lesser toes either side of the suspected web space are passively fully extended on both feet.

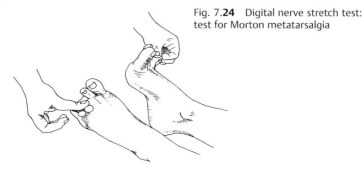

Fig. 7.**24**   Digital nerve stretch test: test for Morton metatarsalgia

**Assessment:**  The test is positive if the patient complains of discomfort in the web space of the affected foot and indicative of Morton meta-tarsalgia.

## Heel Compression Test

Assesses a stress fracture of the calcaneus.

**Procedure:**  The examiner symmetrically compresses the patient's heel between the balls of both thumbs.

**Assessment:**  In a stress fracture of the calcaneus, the patient will feel intense pain in the heel. Stress fractures of the calcaneus primarily occur in patients with significant osteoporosis. Patients with these fractures exhibit a conspicuous antalgic gait, often without any weight bearing on the heel at all. The heel itself may exhibit diffuse swelling and tenderness to palpation. The heel compression test rarely causes serious pain in patients with heel pain from other causes such as retrocalcaneal bursitis.

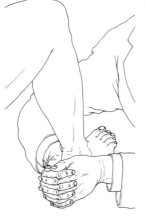

Fig. 7.**25**    Heel compression test

## Tinel Sign

Indicates a tarsal tunnel syndrome.

**Procedure:**  The patient is prone with the knee flexed 90°. The examiner taps the tibial nerve posterior to the medial malleolus with a reflex hammer.

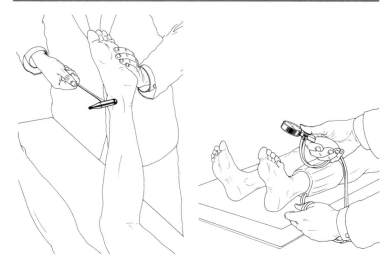

Fig. 7.**26**   Tinel sign                    Fig. 7.**27**   Tourniquet sign

**Assessment:**  Pain and discomfort in the sole of the foot suggest a tarsal tunnel syndrome. This disorder involves chronic neuropathy at the medial malleolus beneath the flexor retinaculum. The nerve can be palpated posterior to the medial malleolus, which will elicit pain. Advanced neuropathy is associated with sensory deficits in the regions supplied by the plantar nerves and paresthesia and atrophy in the plantar muscles.

## Tourniquet Sign

Indicates a tarsal tunnel syndrome.

**Procedure:**  The patient is supine. A blood pressure cuff is applied superior to the malleoli and pumped up above the systolic pressure.

**Assessment:**  Pain and discomfort in the sole of the foot occurring after the pressure has been maintained for a minute indicate compression neuropathy of the tibial nerve at the medial malleolus.

# 8 Posture Deficiency

Rigid erect posture is not only defined by the position of the spine—or trunk—but is primarily the result of muscular activity. We differentiate between rigid erect posture and relaxed erect posture. By rigid erect posture we mean a tense attitude of readiness characterized by a balance in the forces within the musculature, whereas relaxed posture is a lax attitude. This relaxed posture is usually a habitual posture or is characteristic of the individual and depends largely on the individual's particular spinal and pelvic anatomy.

Postural weakness may be defined as extreme difficulty in achieving and maintaining rigid erect posture. The patient is either unable to shift from a relaxed posture to a rigid erect posture or only able to maintain the rigid erect posture temporarily. Chronic postural weakness can lead to degeneration of posture and eventually to a chronic deformity. Postural weakness and degeneration of posture define a continuum, and it is important to promptly identify children and adolescents who are at risk in order to prevent the development of a postural deformity. Posture depends on the quality of the musculature and the existing anatomy. Various functional deviations from the physiologic curvatures have been described. According to Wagenhaeuser, they represent deficient variations of normal posture. These include unsteady posture, round back, sway back, flat back, and lateral deformities.

A differential diagnosis must consider functional postural deficiencies due to spinal disorders such as Scheuermann disease and spondylolisthesis. A variety of posture tests can be used to assess postural deficiencies.

The Matthiass postural competence test allows assessment of the competence of the postural muscles. The Kraus-Weber test allows assessment of the competence of the trunk and pelvic muscles. The strength and endurance of the muscles of the abdomen and back are measured. This test aids in determining the quantitative and qualitative effect of muscular action in neutralizing the effect of the body's weight.

## Kraus–Weber Tests

Test the competence of the trunk and pelvic muscles.

**Procedure: A:**   The patient is supine with the legs and feet extended and the hands clasped behind the head. The patient is then asked to raise his or her extended legs 25 cm and to hold them at this height for 10 seconds. This tests the lower abdominal muscles. It counts 10 points.

**B:**   The patient is supine with the hands clasped behind the head. The examiner immobilizes the patient's feet. The patient is asked to sit up. This tests the upper abdominal muscles. Sitting up 90° counts 10 points; sitting up 45° counts 5 points.

**C:**   The patient is supine with the hands clasped behind the head but with the legs flexed. The examiner immobilizes the patient's feet. The patient is asked to sit up. This tests all of the abdominal muscles with the effect of the psoas neutralized.

**D:**   The patient is prone with a cushion beneath the abdomen and hands clasped behind the head. The examiner immobilizes the patient's hips and feet against the examining table. The patient is asked to raise his or her body off the examining table and to maintain that position for 10 seconds. This tests the upper back muscles. It counts 10 points.

**E:**   The patient is prone with a cushion beneath the pelvis. The examiner immobilizes the patient's trunk and hips against the examining table. The patient is asked to raise his or her legs off the examining table with the feet extended and to maintain that position for 10 seconds. This tests the lower back muscles. It counts 10 points.

**F:**   The patient stands barefoot with hands at his or her sides. The patient is then asked to bend over with the knees extended and arms stretched out in front. The examiner measures the distance to the floor.

**Assessment:**   Normal results for the Kraus-Weber test are indicated by this index:

$$A\,\frac{10}{10} \qquad B\,\frac{10}{10} \qquad FBA = 0$$

where A represents the strength of the abdominal muscles and B the strength of the back muscles. The numerators are the values for the upper abdominal muscles and upper back muscles, respectively; the denominators are the values for the lower abdominal muscles and lower back muscles including the psoas, respectively.

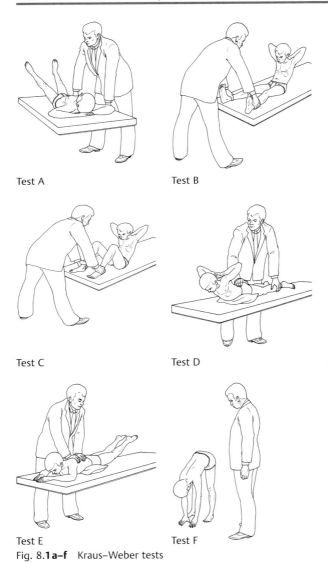

Test A

Test B

Test C

Test D

Test E

Test F

Fig. 8.**1 a–f**   Kraus–Weber tests

## Matthiass Postural Competence Tests

Assess the competence of the back and trunk muscles in children and adolescents.

**Procedure:**   The examination is performed with the patient standing. The child is asked to lift the arms and keep them in that position.

**Assessment:**   Raising the arms shifts the body's center of gravity forward.

The child with normal posture compensates for the shift in the center of gravity by leaning the entire body slightly backward. A child with postural weakness will exhibit increased thoracic kyphosis and lumbar lordosis.

Matthiass identifies two degrees of postural weakness.

Patients with full muscular function will usually be able to achieve and maintain full erect posture with minimal backward bending in the arm-raising test. In first-degree postural weakness, the child can actively achieve full erect posture but within 30 seconds slumps into a backward bending posture with increased thoracic kyphosis and lumbar lordosis.

Second-degree postural weakness is where the child is unable to actively achieve full erect posture and slumps backward right at the start of the arm-raising test. The child will push the pelvis forward and greatly increase the lumbar lordosis. This is referred to as postural degeneration.

The differential diagnosis must include functional postural deficits due to organic spinal disorders. A thorough clinical examination with function tests will allow postural weakness to be distinguished from deformities and idiopathic disorders at an early stage. In particular, examination must exclude scoliosis and kyphosis, as well as deformities such as flat back, round back, or sway back.

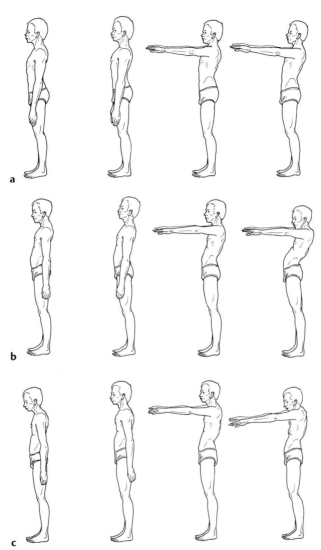

Fig. **8.2a–c**   Matthiass postural competence tests:
**a** normal posture,
**b** postural weakness,
**c** postural degeneration

# 9 Venous Thrombosis

Acute deep venous thrombosis ranks with acute arterial occlusion as one of the most serious and dramatic vascular emergencies. Factors contributing to thrombosis include vessel wall, blood flow, and coagulation characteristics. Thromboses most commonly develop in the lower extremities. They are a feared postoperative complication as they involve the risk of acute massive or recurrent pulmonary embolism. Thrombosis in the deep veins of the leg is less symptomatic yet involves a far greater risk of embolism than thrombosis in the superficial veins. Swelling in the extremity (primarily in the left leg at the vascular spur in the pelvic veins), often associated with spontaneous pain in the groin, and pain radiating into the leg upon coughing or straining, local blue discoloration of the skin, and in some cases elevated temperature and pulse are important signs. However, a pulmonary infarction will often be the first clinical symptom. Yet typical early signs of deep venous thrombosis may also occur. These include spots that are painful to palpation, extending from the sole of the foot (Payr) to, in certain cases, the groin (Rielander), and pain upon compression of the calf (Lowenberg) when a blood pressure cuff is applied and pumped up to 100 mmHg (13.3 kPa). However, these thrombosis signs are nonspecific and should by no means be regarded as conclusive. The unilateral edema that usually occurs develops gradually and begins in the malleolar region. Additional characteristic findings include distended congested peripheral veins in the affected extremity (Pratt "warning" veins), evidence of superficial collateral veins, and an expanding edema.

In patients with chronic venous disease, a number of test methods are helpful in evaluating the function of the deep veins and perforating veins.

## Lowenberg Test

Early sign of venous thrombosis.

**Procedure:**   The examiner applies a blood pressure cuff to each lower leg and pumps them up.

**Assessment:**   Normally, discomfort will occur only beyond 180 mmHg (24 kPa). Where thrombosis is present, the normal leg will be observed to tolerate compression of the calf musculature with far higher pressure than the affected leg.

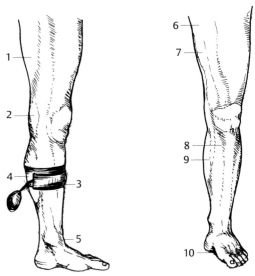

Fig. **9.1a, b**   Early signs of deep venous thrombosis:
1 Tenderness to palpation on the medial aspect of the thigh (sartorius, gracilis)
2 Tenderness to palpation in the knee (muscular insertions and medial joint cavity)
3 Pain on compression of the calf (Lowenberg)
4 Pain in the calf on dorsiflexion of the foot (Homans sign)
5 Tenderness to palpation
6 Groin pain
7 Tenderness to palpation along the adductors
8 Pratt warning sign
9 Meyer pressure points along the great saphenous vein
10 Pain in the sole of the foot, Payr sign upon pressing or tapping the sole of the foot with the edge of the hand

## Trendelenburg Test

Assesses varicose veins in the thigh. Tests the function of the lesser saphenous vein and perforating veins.

**Procedure:** With the patient supine and the leg raised, the examiner smoothes the distended veins. The examiner then compresses the greater saphenous vein with a tourniquet distal to its junction with the femoral vein at the inguinal ligament and asks the patient to stand up.

**Evaluation:** If the varices only fill up slowly or not at all within 30 seconds of the patient standing up but then fill rapidly from proximal once the tourniquet is loosened, this indicates valvular insufficiency of the saphenous vein with normal function of perforating veins. Relatively rapid filling from distal can occur as a result of insufficient perforating veins or anastomoses with an insufficient lesser saphenous vein. Rapid filling of the varices from both distal and proximal once the tourniquet is released indicates insufficiency of both the greater saphenous vein and the communication with the deeper venous system.

## Perthes Test

Assesses the function of deep veins and perforating veins.

**Procedure:** With the patient standing, the examiner applies a tourniquet to the thigh or lower leg proximal to the filled varices. The patient is then asked to walk around with the tourniquet in place.

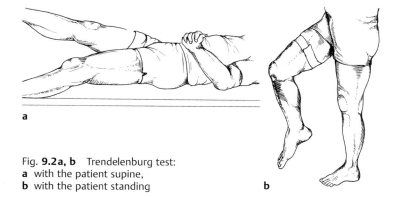

**a**

Fig. **9.2a, b**  Trendelenburg test:
**a**  with the patient supine,
**b**  with the patient standing **b**

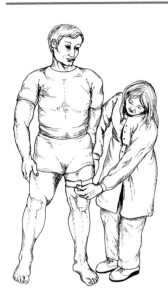

Fig. 9.**3**   Perthes test

**Assessment:**   Complete emptying of the varices as a result of muscular activity indicates proper function of the perforating veins and intact deep venous drainage. The congestion is attributable to valvular insufficiency in the saphenous vein. Incomplete emptying is observed where there is moderate valvular insufficiency of the communicating veins. Unchanged filling in the varices occurs with significant insufficiency of the perforating veins and impaired blood flow in the deep veins. An increase in filling suggests a severe post-thrombotic syndrome with reversed blood flow in the perforating veins.

**Note:**   The Schwartz test or the percussion method of Schwartz and Hackenbruch is used to assess valvular insufficiency in the region of the greater saphenous vein. With the patient standing, the examiner places one finger on the distended vein being examined and taps on the junction of the greater saphenous and femoral veins with one finger of the other hand. If this tapping is transmitted back to the first finger, the blood flow is continuous, indicating that the valves in the portion of the vein being examined are not intact. The test is not necessarily definitive, but it is good method for determining whether a superficial venous branch communicates with the greater or lesser saphenous vein.

## Homans Test

Assesses deep venous thrombosis.

**Procedure:** The patient is supine. The examiner lifts the affected leg and rapidly dorsiflexes the patient's foot with the knee extended. This maneuver is repeated with the patient's knee flexed while the examiner simultaneously palpates the calf.

**Assessment:** Pain occurring upon dorsiflexion of the foot with the knee extended and flexed indicates thrombosis or thrombophlebitis.

Calf pain with the knee extended can also be caused by intervertebral disk disease (radicular symptoms) or muscle contractures.

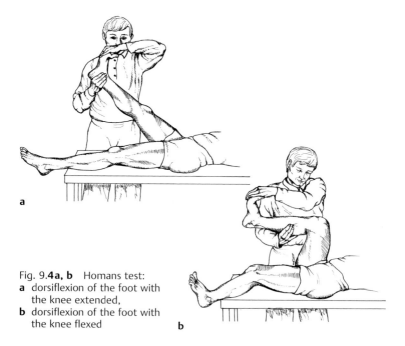

Fig. 9.**4a, b** Homans test:
**a** dorsiflexion of the foot with the knee extended,
**b** dorsiflexion of the foot with the knee flexed

# 10 Occlusive Arterial Disease

Occlusive arterial disease is often associated with orthopedic disorders. Notably, nearly 90% of all cases of obliterative arteriosclerosis involve exclusively the lower extremities. Prior to treating the actual orthopedic disorder, the physician must take care to exclude or identify any possible arterial ischemic disorders. After obtaining a detailed history, a diagnosis can usually be made on the basis of inspection, palpation, and specific function tests, and usually will not require the use of any diagnostic technology.

Weakened or absent arterial pulse, cool and pale skin (or cyanotic skin), patches of erythema, and trophic disturbances are signs of occlusive arterial disease. Ulceration and gangrene are signs of advanced disease. Where typical symptoms of intermittent claudication (calf pain after walking short distances) are present, determining the maximum distance the patient can walk without experiencing these symptoms can help in estimating the severity of the disorder (Fontaine classification of the severity of occlusive arterial disease). The differential diagnosis of intermittent claudication must include spinal claudication from compression of the cauda equina, the cardinal symptom of lumbar spinal stenosis. The intermittent claudication in cauda equina pathology is not a sharply defined clinical syndrome. Radicular symptoms such as paresthesia, pain, sensory deficits, and weakness can occur in one or both legs when the patient stands or walks. These symptoms may improve or disappear when the patient stops moving, as in the vascular form, but more often will do so only on certain body movements.

**Note:** The walking test allows assessment of peripheral circulatory disruption. The patient is asked to walk up and down a long corridor for up to three minutes at about 120 paces per minute. The time of occurrence of symptoms and the site of pain are clinically assessed, as are gait and any pauses. If the patient pauses after only 60 seconds, this suggests disruption of vascular supply to the muscles. Symptoms of moderately severe circulatory disruption will manifest themselves after 1–3 minutes of walking. Symptoms that occur only after three minutes or more of walking indicate only slight circulatory disruption.

Note that exercise tolerance may be limited by cardiac and pulmonary disorders as well as orthopedic disorders such as osteoarthritis of the hip or degenerative knee disorders.

## Allen Test

Assesses an arterial ischemic disorder in the upper extremities.

**Procedure:**   The patient is seated and raises his or her arm above the horizontal plane. The examiner grasps the patient's wrist and applies finger pressure to block the vascular supply from the radial and ulnar arteries. The patient then makes a fist so as to force the venous blood out of the hand via the posterior veins. After one minute, the patient lets the arm hang down and opens the now pale hand. The examiner simultaneously releases compression, first from one artery then from the other.

**Evaluation:**   Rapid, uniform reddening of the hand in the areas supplied by the respective arteries indicates normal arterial supply. If vascular supply to the hand and fingers is compromised, the ischemic changes in the hand will only slowly recede.

## George Vertebral Artery Test (De Klyn Test)

Assessment of vertebral, basilar, or carotid artery stenosis or compression.

**Procedure:**   This test requires certain preliminary findings as it is not entirely without risk. Parameters requiring prior assessment include blood pressure, arm pulse, and pulses in the common carotid and subclavian arteries with auscultation to detect any murmurs or bruits. This test should not be performed if any of these prior examinations produces significantly abnormal findings. In the absence of any significant abnormalities, the seated patient is asked to maximally rotate his or her head to one side while extending the neck. The test can also be performed with the patient supine, in which case the patient's head projects over the edge of the examining table and rests in the examiner's hands. Then with the head hanging down (in the De Klyn position), the head is maximally rotated and the neck extended. The head should

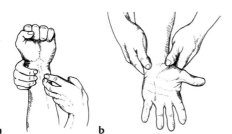

Fig. 10.**1a, b**   Allen test:
**a** palpation of vessels with the arm raised,
**b** palpation of vessels with the arm hanging and evaluation of skin perfusion

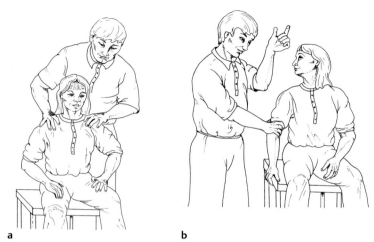

a                                    b

Fig. 10.**2a, b**   George vertebral artery test:
**a** starting position,
**b** rotation of the head and extension of the cervical spine

remain or be held in maximum rotation and extension for about 20–30 seconds. The patient is then requested to count out loud.

**Assessment:**   Abnormal auscultatory findings in the common carotid artery, vertigo, visual symptoms, nausea, fatigue, or nystagmus occurring during this maximum rotation and extension indicate stenosis of the vertebral artery or common carotid artery. The test is especially important in candidates for treatment (such as traction or manipulative therapy) of cervical spine symptoms associated with vertigo. The vertebral artery provocation test aids in the differential diagnosis because nausea, vertigo, and nystagmus initially increase but then rapidly decrease in intensity where a vertebral blockade is present. In the presence of vertebral artery insufficiency, the intensity of nausea and vertigo symptoms will rapidly increase within a few seconds without abating.

### Ratschow-Boerger Test

Assessment of vascular disease in the pelvis and legs.

**Procedure:**   The supine patient is asked to raise the legs as high as possible and continuously rotate or plantar flex and dorsiflex the feet.

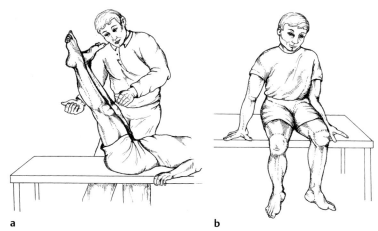

**a**                                    **b**

Fig. 10.**3a, b**   Ratschow–Boerger test:
**a** patient supine with the legs raised
**b** patient sitting with the legs hanging down over the edge of the examining
   table

**Assessment:**   Patients with normal vascular function will be able to perform this maneuver without any pain and without the soles of the feet becoming pale. Patients with compromised vascular function will experience varying degrees of pain and significant ischemia in the sole of the foot on the affected side. After about two minutes, the patient is requested to sit up quickly and let the legs hang over the edge of the examining table. Reactive hyperemia and refilling of the veins will occur within 5–7 seconds in patients with normal vascular function. In patients with compromised vascular function, this reaction will be delayed in proportion to the severity of vascular stenosis.

## ▉   Thoracic Outlet Syndrome

Thoracic outlet syndrome is a compression syndrome at the base of the neck with compromised neurovascular function. Thoracic outlet syndrome can be a congenital disorder resulting from factors such as a cervical rib, a superiorly displaced first rib, atypical ligaments, and the presence of an atypical small scalene muscle. It may also be acquired as a result of callus formation, osteophytes on the clavicle and first rib, and changes in the scalene muscles such as fibrosis or hypertrophy.

This syndrome may be further differentiated according to the compression site as a cervical rib syndrome, first-rib syndrome, or scalene muscle syndrome. For this reason, a diagnosis of thoracic outlet syndrome is usually one of exclusion in which all other causes have been eliminated.

### Costoclavicular Test

Assesses a neurovascular compression syndrome in the costoclavicular region.

**Procedure:**  The patient is seated with the arms hanging relaxed. The examiner palpates the wrists to take the pulse in both radial arteries, noting amplitude and pulse rate. Then the patient abducts and externally both arms and retracts the shoulders. With the patient in this position, the examiner again palpates the wrists and evaluates the pulse in both radial arteries.

**Assessment:**  Unilateral weakness or absence of the pulse in the radial artery, ischemic skin changes, and paresthesia are clear signs of compression of the neurovascular bundle in the costoclavicular region (between the first rib and clavicle).

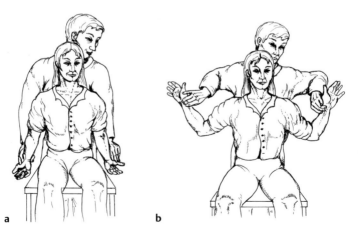

Fig. 10.**4a, b**  Costoclavicular test:
**a** starting position with the examiner palpating the pulse in the radial arteries,
**b** palpation of the pulse in the radial arteries in abduction, with arms externally rotated and shoulders retracted

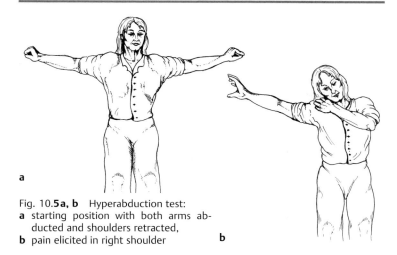

Fig. 10.**5a, b** Hyperabduction test:
**a** starting position with both arms abducted and shoulders retracted,
**b** pain elicited in right shoulder

## Hyperabduction Test

Indicates a scalene muscle syndrome.

**Procedure:** The standing patient abducts both arms past 90° while retracting the shoulders. Then the patient opens each hand and makes a fist with each hand for two minutes.

**Assessment:** Pain in the shoulder and arm, ischemic skin changes, and paresthesia are clear signs of compression of the neurovascular bundle, which is primarily attributable to changes in the scalene muscles (fibrosis, hypertrophy, or presence of a small scalene muscle).

### Intermittent Claudication Test

Sign of a costoclavicular compression syndrome.

**Procedure:** The standing patient abducts and externally rotates both arms. Then the patient is instructed to rapidly flex and extend the fingers of each hand for one minute.

**Assessment:** If one arm begins to droop after a few cycles of finger motion and ischemic skin changes, paresthesia, and pain in the shoulder and arm occur, this suggests a costoclavicular compression syndrome affecting neurovascular structures.

Causes include osteophytes, rib changes, and anatomic variations in the scalene muscles.

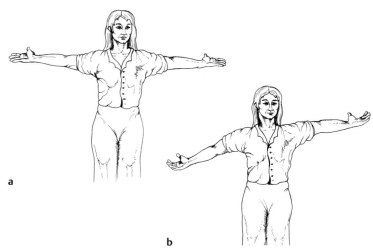

Fig. 10.**6a, b**    Intermittent claudication test:
**a** starting position with both arms abducted and externally rotated,
**b** pain on the right side with drooping right arm

## Adson Test

**Procedure:**    The patient's head is rotated to face the test shoulder. He or she then extends the head while the examiner externally rotates and extends the shoulder. The examiner locates the radial pulse and the patient is instructed to take a deep breath and hold it.

**Assessment:**    A disappearance of the pulse indicates a positive test. The test is significant for identifying neurovascular compression of the sub-clavian artery and brachial plexus of the ipsilateral side, which are commonly caused by scalenus anticus or cervical rib thoracic outlet syndromes.

## Allen Maneuver

Indicates a thoracic outlet syndrome.

**Procedure:**    The patient is sitting or standing. The examiner is standing behind the patient. He flexes the patient's elbow to 90° while the shoulder is abducted horizontally and placed into external rotation. The patient then rotates the head away from the test side.

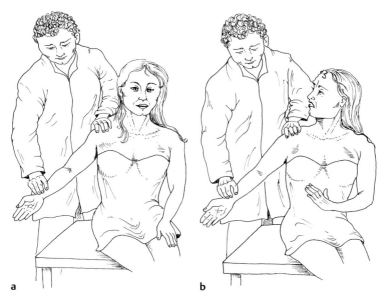

Fig. 10.**7a, b** Adson test:
**a** starting position,
**b** the patient rotates toward the affected shoulder and extends the head

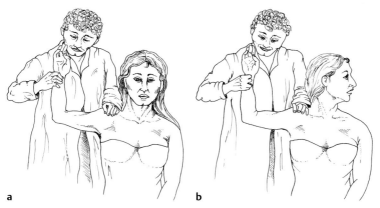

Fig. 10.**8a, b** Allen maneuver:
**a** starting position,
**b** the patient rotates the head to the opposite side

**Assessment:**  The examiner palpates the radial pulse which disappears when the head is rotated.

This disappearance indicates a positive test result for thoracic outlet syndrome (e. g., clavicular fractures with excessive callus or residual displacements of fragments, a cervical rib, a bifid clavicle, abnormal splitting of the scalenus medius may contribute to compression symptoms).

**Note:** Hyperabducting the arm so that the hand is brought over the head with the elbow arm in the coronal plane with the shoulder laterally rotated is a maneuver called the Wright test. The pulse is palpated for differences.

## ▇ Hemiparesis

### Arm-Holding Test

Assessment of latent hemiparesis.

**Procedure:**  The patient is asked to supinate both arms and raise them to 90° while keeping his or her eyes closed.

**Assessment:**  Pronation and a drop in one arm suggest latent central hemiparesis. Where the arm first drops and then pronates with the patient's eyes closed, one should consider psychogenic influence.

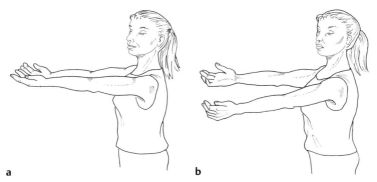

a                                    b

Fig. 10.**9a, b**   Arm holding test:
**a** Both arms supinated and raised up to 90° with closed eyes,
**b** Pronation and drop in one arm

## Leg-Holding Test

Assessment of latent central hemiparesis.

**Procedure:**   The patient is supine and is asked to close his or her eyes and flex both hips and both knees. The examiner watches the lower legs to see if they drop down.

**Assessment:**   The neurologic examination of the lower extremities in a patient capable of standing and walking begins with inspection of gait. The patient is asked to stand and walk on tiptoe and then on his or her heels. This will usually exclude any gross motor deficits. With the patient supine, the strength of the quadriceps is then tested by having the patient extend the knee against the examiner's resistance (L3–L4). Strength in the extensor digitorum and hallucis longus is tested by dorsiflexion of the toes (L5) against resistance, and strength in the triceps surae is tested by plantar flexion of the foot (S1) against resistance. One or both lower legs dropping down during the leg holding test can be a sign of latent central hemiparesis.

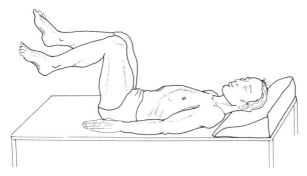

Fig. 10.**10**   Leg holding test

# References

## Spine—Sacroiliac Joint

Andersson GBJ, Deyo RA. History and physical examination in patients with herniated lumbar discs. Spine. 1996;21:10S–18 S.

Baker S, Kesson M, Ashmore J, Turner G, Conway J, Stevens D. Guidance for pre-manipulative testing of the cervical spine. Man Ther. 2000;5:37–40.

Bland JH. Disorders of the Cervical Spine. Philadelphia: WB Saunders Co;1994.

Borge JA, Leboeuf-Yde C, Lothe J. Prognostic values for physical examination findings in patients with chronic low back pain treated conservatively: A systematic literature review. J Manip Physiol Ther. 2001;24:292–295.

Cameron DM, Bohannon RW, Owen SV. Influence of hip position on measurements of straight leg raise test. J Orthop Sports Phys Ther. 1994;19:168–172.

Childs JD. One on one: The impact of the Valsalva maneuver during resistance exercise. Strength and Conditioning Journal. 1999;21:54–55.

Christodoulides AN. Ipsilateral sciatica on femoral nerve stretch test is pathognomonic of an L4/5 disk protrusion. J Bone Joint Surg Br. 1989;71:88–89.

Devereaux MW. Neck and low back pain. Med Clin North Am. 2003;87:643–662.

Deville WL, Van der Windt DA, Dzaferagic A, Bezemer PD, Bouter LM. The test of Lasegue: Systematic review of the accuracy in diagnosing herniated discs. Spine. 2000;25:1140–1147.

Dobbs, AC. Evaluation of instabilities of the lumbar spine. Orthop Phys Ther Clin North Am. 1999;8:387–400.

Dreyfuss PH, Michaelsen M, Pauza M, McLarty J, Bogduk N. The value of history and physical examination in diagnosing sacroiliac joint pain. Spine. 1996;2594–2602.

Dvorak J. Neurophysiologic tests in diagnosis of nerve root compression caused by disc herniation. Spine. 1996;21:39S–44 S.

Dvorak J, Antinnes JA, Panjabi M, Loustalot D, Bonomo M. Age and gender related normal motion of the cervical spine. Spine. 1992;17:S 393–S 398.

Dyck P. The femoral nerve traction test with lumbar disc protrusion. Surg Neurol. 1976;6:163–166.

Elvey RL. The investigation of arm pain. In: Boyling JD, Palastanga N, eds. Grieve's Modern Manual Therapy: The Vertebral Column. 2nd ed. Edinburgh: Churchill Livingstone;1994.

Evans R, ed. Cervical spine. In: Evans R, ed. Illustrated Orthopaedic Physical Assessment.2nd ed. St. Louis: CV Mosby Co;2001.

Fast A, Parikh S, Marin EL. The shoulder abduction relief sign in cervical radiculopathy. Arch Phys Med Rehabil. 1989;87:402–403.

Ginsberg GM, Bassett GS. Back pain in children and adolescents: Evaluation and differential diagnosis. J Am Acad Orthop Surg. 1997;5:67–78.

Hall TM, Elvey RL. Nerve trunk pain: Physical diagnosis and treatment. Man Ther. 1999;4:63–73.

Hoover CF. A new sign for the detection of malingering and functional paresis of the lower extremities. JAMA. 1908;51:746–747.

Hourigan CL, Bassett JM. Facet syndrome: Clinical signs, symptoms, diagnosis, and treatment. J Manip Physiol Ther. 1989;12:293–297.

Johnson EK, Chiarello CM. The slump test: The effects of head and lower extremity position on knee extension. J Orthop Sports Phys Ther. 1997;26:310–317.

Jonsson B, Strömqvist B. The straight leg raising test and the severity of symptoms in lumbar disc herniation: A preoperative evaluation. Spine. 1995;20:27–30.

Kleinrensink GJ, Stoeckart R, Mulder PG, et al. Upper limb tension tests as tolls in the diagnosis of nerve and plexus lesions: Anatomical and biochemical aspects. Clin Biochem (Bristol, Avon). 2000;15:9–14.

Koehler PJ, Okun MS. Important observations prior to the description of the Hoover sign. Neurology. 2004;63:1693–1697.

Laslett M, Young SB, Aprill CN, McDonald B. Diagnosing painful sacroiliac joints: A validity study of a McKenzie evaluation and sacroiliac provocation tests. Australian Journal of Physiotherapy. 2003;49:89–97.

Lee DG. Rotational instability of the midthoracic spine: Assessment and management. Man Ther. 1996;1:234–241.

Lew PC, Briggs CA. Relationship between the cervical component of the slump test and change in hamstring muscle tension. Man Ther. 1997;2:98–110.

Maitland GD. The slump test: Examination and treatment. Aust J Physiother. 1985;31:215–219.

Malanga G, Landes P, Nadler SF. Provocative tests in cervical spine examination: Historical basis and scientific analyses. Pain Physician. 2003;6:199–205.

Mitchell J, Keene D, Dyson C, Harvey L, Pruvey C, Phillips R. Is cervical spine rotation, as used in the standard vertebrobasilar insufficiency test, associated with a measurable change in intracranial vertebral artery blood flow? Man Ther. 2004;9:220–227.

Nilsson N, Hartvigsen J, Christensen HW. Normal ranges of passive cervical motion for women and men 20–60 years old. J Manip Physiol Ther. 1996;19:306–309.

Rubinstein SM, Pool JJ, Van Tulder MW, Riphagen II, De Vet HC. A systematic review of the diagnostic accuracy of provocative tests of the neck for diagnosing cervical radiculopathy. Eur Spine J. 2007;16:307–319.

Sandmark H, Nisell R. Validity of five common manual neck pain provoking tests. Scand J Rehabil Med. 1995;27:131–136.

Shacklock MO. Positive upper limp tension test in a case of surgically proven neuropathy: Analysis and validity. Man Ther. 1996;1:154–161.

Shah KC, Rajshekhar V. Reliability of diagnosis of soft cervical disc prolapse using Spurling's test. Br J Neurosurg. 2004;18:480–483.

Spurling RG, Scoville WB. Lateral rupture of the cervical intervertebral discs: A common cause of shoulder and arm pain. Surg Gynecol Obstet. 1944;78:350–358.

Sullivan MS, Schoaf LD, Riddle DL. The relationship of lumbar flexion to disability in patients with low back pain. Phys Ther. 2000;80:240–250.

Supik LF, Broom MJ. Sciatic tension signs and lumbar disc herniation. Spine. 1994;19(9):1066–9

Thomas KE, Hasbun R, Jekel J, Quagliarello VJ. The diagnostic accuracy of Kernig's sign, Brudzinski's sign, and nuchal rigidity in adults with suspected meningitis. Clinical Infectious Diseases. 2002;35:46–52.

Tong HC, Haig AJ, Yamakawa K. The Spurling test and cercial radiculopathy. Spine. 2002;27:156–159.

Torg JS, Ramsey-Emrhein JA. Cervical spine and brachial plexus injuries: Return to play recommendation. Phys Sportsmed. 1997;25: 61–88.

Walch MJ. Evaluation of orthopaedic testing of the low back for non-specific low back pain. J Manip Physiol Ther. 1998;21:232–236.

Wartenberg R. The signs of Brudzinski and of Kernig. J Pediatr. 1950;37:679–684.

White MA, Pape KE. The slump test. Am J Occup Ther. 1992;46:271–274.

Worth DR. Movements of the head and neck. In: Boyling JD, Palastanga N, eds. Grieve's Manual Therapy: The Vertebral Column. 2nd ed. Edinburgh: Churchill Livingstone;1994.

Youdas JW, Garrett TR, Suman VJ, Bogard CL, Hallman HO, Carey JR. Normal range of motion of the cervical spine: An initial goniometric study. Phys Ther. 1992;72:770–780.

Young S, Aprill C. Characteristics of a mechanical assessment for chronic lumbar facet joint pain. J Man Manip Ther.2000;8:78–84

Young S, Aprill C, Laslett M. Correlation of clinical examination characteristics with three sources of chronic low back pain. The Spine Journal. 2003;3:460–465.

Zaina C, Grant R, Johnson C, Dansie B, Taylor J, Spyropolous P. The effect of cervical rotation on blood flow in the contralateral vertebral artery. Man Ther. 2003;8:103–109.

Zito G, Jull G, Story I. Clinical tests of musculoskeletal dysfunction in the diagnosis of cervicogenic headache. Man Ther. 2006;11:118–129.

## Shoulder

Berg EE, Ciullo JV. A clinical test for superior glenoid labral or superior labrum anterior-posterior (SLAP) lesions. Clin J Sport Med. 1998;8:121–123.

Calis M, Akgün K, Birtane M, Karacan I, Calis H, Tuzun F. Diagnostic values of clinical diagnostic tests in subacromial impingement syndrome. Ann Rheum Dis. 2000;59:44–47.

Chronopoulus E., Kim TK, Park HB, Ashenbrenner D, McFarland EG. Diagnostic value of physical tests for isolated chronic AC lesions. Am J Sports Med. 2004;32:655–661.

De Wilde L, Plasschaert F, Berghs B, Van Hoecke M, Verstraete K, Verdonk R. Quantified measurement of subacromial impingement. J Shoulder Elbow Surg. 2003;12:346–349.

Emery RJ, Mullaji AB. Glenohumeral joint instability in normal adolescents: Incidence and significance. J Bone Joint Surg Br. 1991;73:406–408.

Gagey OJ, Gagey N. The hyperabduction test: An assessment of the laxity of the inferior glenohumeral ligament. J Bone Joint Surg Br. 2001;83B:69–74.

Gerber C, Ganz R. Clinical assessment of instability of the shoulder with special reference to anterior and posterior drawer tests. J Bone Joint Surg Br. 1984;66B:551–556.

Guanche CA, Jones DC. Clinical testing for tears of the glenoid labrum. Arthroscopy. 2003;19:517–523.

Hawkins RJ, Bokor DJ. Clinical evaluation of shoulder problems. In: Rockwood CA, Matsen FA III, eds. The Shoulder. Vol 1. Philadelphia: WB Saunders;1990:pp 149–177.

Hawkins RJ, Kennedy JC. Impingement syndrome in athletes. Am J Sports Med. 1980;8:151–158.

Hertel R, Ballmer FT, Lambert SM, Gerber C. Lag signs in the diagnosis of rotator cuff rupture. J Shoulder Elbow Surg. 1996;5:307–313.

Ide M, Ide J, Yamaga M, Takagi K. Symptoms and signs of irritation of the brachial plexus in whiplash injuries. Bone Joint Surg (Br). 2001;83B:226–229.

Jensen C, Rayan GM. Thoracic outlet syndrome: Provocative examination maneuvers in a typical population. J Shoulder Elbow Surg. 1995;4:113–117.

Kelly JJ. Neurological problems in the athlete's shoulder. In: Pettrone FA, ed. Athletic Injuries of the Shoulder. New York: McGraw-Hill;1995.

Kim SH, Park JC, Park JS, Oh I. Painful jerk test: A predictor of success in nonoperative treatment of painful inferior instability of the shoulder. Am J Sports Med. 2004;32:1849–1855.

Kirkley A, Litchfield RB, Jackowski DM, Lo IK. The use of the impingement test as a predictor of outcome following subacromial decompression for rotator cuff tendinosis. Arthroscopy. 2002;18:8–15.

Kirkley A, Nonweiler B, Lo IKY, Woolfrey M. Validation of the apprehension relocation and surprise tests in the diagnosis of anterior shoulder instability. J Bone Joint Surg (Br). 1997;79B:75.

Kolbel, R. A modification of the relocation test: Arthroscopic findings associated with a positive test. J Shoulder Elbow Surg. 2001;10:497–498.

Koslow, PA, Prosser LA, Strony GA, Suchecki SL, Mattingly GE. Specificity of the lateral scapular slide test in asymptomatic competitive athletes. J Orthop Sports Phys Ther. 2003;33:331–336.

Limb D. How I examine the shoulder: A guide from the expert. Current Orthopaedics. 2000;14:435–440.

Lo IK, Nonweiler B, Woolfrey M, Litchfield R, Kirkley A. An evaluation of the apprehension, relocation and surprise tests for anterior shoulder instability. Am J Sports Med. 2004;32:301–307.

Ludington NA. Rupture of the long head of the biceps flexor cubiti muscle. Ann Surg. 1923;77:358–363.

MacDonald PB, Clark P, Sutherland K. An analysis of the diagnostic accuracy of the Hawkins and Neer subacromial impingement signs. J Shoulder Elbow Surg. 2000;9:299–301.

McFarland EG, Kim TK, Savino RM. Clinical assessment of three common tests for superior labral anterior-posterior lesions. Am J Sports Med. 2002;30:810–815.

Meister K, Buckley B, Batts J. The posterior impingement sign: Diagnosis of rotator cuff and posterior labral tears secondary to internal impingement in overhead athletes. Am J Orthop. 2004;33:412–415.

Mimori K, Muneta T, Nakagawa T, Shinomiya K. A new pain provocation test for superior labral tears of the shoulder. Am J Sports Med. 1999;27:137–142.

Neer CS. Anterior acromioplasty for the chronic impingement syndrome in the shoulder. J Bone Joiunt Surg Am. 1972;54A:41.

O'Brien SJ, Pagnani MJ, Fealy S, McGlynn SR, Wilson JB. The active compression test: A new and effective test for diagnosing labral tears and acromioclavicular joint abnormality. Am J Sports Med. 1998;26:610–613.

Park, HB, Yokota A, Gill HS, El Rassi G, McFarland EG. Diagnostic accuracy of clinical tests for the different degrees of subacromial impingement syndrome. Bone Joint Surg Am. 2005;87:1446–1455.

Plewa MC, Delinger M. The false-positive rate of thoracic outlet syndrome shoulder maneuvers in healthy subjects. Acad Emerg Med. 1998;5:337–342.

Rockwood CA, Matsen FA. The Shoulder. Vol 1. 2nd ed. Philadelphia: WB Saunders;1998.

Stetson WB, Templin K. The crank test, the O'Brien test, and routine magnetic resonance imaging scans in the diagnosis of labral tears. Am J Sport Med. 2002;30:806–809.

Tzannes A, Paxinos A, Callanan M, Murrell GA. An assessment of the interexaminer reliability of tests for shoulder instability. J Shoulder Elbow Surg. 2004;13:18–23.

Valadie AL 3 rd., Jobe CM, Pink MM, Ekman EF, Jobe FW. Anatomy of provocative tests for impingement syndrome of the shoulder. J Shoulder Elbow Surg. 2000;9:36–46.

Walch G, Boulahia A, Calderone S, Robinson AHN. The "dropping" and "hornblower's" signs in evaluation of rotator cuff tears. J Bone Joint Surg (Br). 1998;73B:624–628.

Yergason RM. Supination sign. J Bone Joint Surg. 1931;13:160.

## Elbow

Alfonso MI, Dzwierzynski W. Tinel's sign: The realities. Phys Med Rehabil Clin N Am. 1998;9:721–736.

Anderson TE. Anatomy and physical examination of the elbow. In: Nicholas JA, Hershmann EB, eds. The Upper Extremity in Sports Medicine. St. Louis: CV Mosby Co;1990.

Andrews JR, Wilk KE, Satterwhite YE, et al. Physical examination of the thrower's elbow. J Orthop Sports Phys Ther. 1993;17:296–304.

Buehler MJ, Thayer DT. The elbow flexion test: A clinical test for the cubital tunnel syndrome. Clin Orthop. 1988;233:213–216.

Cohen MS, Hastings H. Rotatory instability of the elbow: The anatomy and role of the lateral stabilizers. J Bone Joint Surg Am. 1997;79:225–233.

Landi A, Copeland S. Value of the Tinel sign in brachial plexus lesions. Ann R Coll Surg Engl. 1979;61:470–471.

Leach RE, Miller JK. Lateral and medial epicondylitis of the elbow. Clin Sports Med. 1987;6:259–272.

Lee ML, Rosenwasser MP. Chronic elbow instability. Orthop Clin North Am.1999;30:81–89.

MacDermid JC, Michlovitz SL. Examination of the elbow: Linking diagnosis, prognosis and outcomes as a framework for maximizing therapy interventions. J Hand Ther. 2006;19:82–97.

McGall BR, Cain EL. Diagnosis, treatment, and rehabilitation of the thrower's elbow. Curr Sports Med Rep.2005;4:249–254.

McPherson SA, Meals RA. Cubital tunnel syndrome. Orthop Clin.North Am. 1992;23:111–123.

Mehta JA, Bain GI. Posterolateral rotatory instability of the elbow. J Am Acad Orthop Surg. 2004;12:405–415.

Morrey BF. Acute and chronic instability of the elbow. J Am Acad Orthop Surg. 1996;4:117–128.

Novak CB, Gilbert WL, Mackinnon SE, Lay L. Provocative testing for cubital tunnel syndrome. J Hand Surg. 1994;19A:817–820.

O'Driscoll SW. Classification and evaluation of recurrent instability of the elbow. Clin Orthop.2000;370:34–43.

O'Driscoll SW, Bell DF, Morrey BF. Posterolateral rotatory instability of the elbow. J Bone Joint Surg. 1991;73A:440–446.

Phalen GS. The carpal-tunnel-syndrome: Clinical evaluation of 598 hands. Clin Orthop.1972;83:29–40.

Plancher KD, Halbrecht J, Lourie GM. Medial and lateral epicondylitis in the athlete. Clin Sports Med. 1996;15:283–303.

Rayan GM, Jensen C, Duke J. Elbow flexion test in the normal population. J Hand Surg. 1992;17A:86–89.

## Hand

Bechtal CD. The use of a dynamometer with adjustable handle spacing.J Bone Joint Surg. 1954;36:820–832.

Bednar JM, Osterman AL. Carpal instability: Evaluation and treatment. J Am Acad Orthop Surg.1993;1:10–17.

Bickert B, Sauerbier M, Germann G. Clinical examination of the injured wrist. (Trans). Zentralbl Chir. 1997;122:1010–1015.

Bozek M, Gazdzik TS. The value of clinical examination in the diagnosis of carpal tunnel syndrome. Ortop Traumatol Rehabil. 2001;3:357–360.

Brüske J, Bednarski M, Grzelec H, Zyluk A. The usefulness of the Phalen test and the Hoffmann-Tinel sign in the diagnosis of carpal tunnel syndrome. Acta Orthop Belg. 2002;68:141–145.

Buch-Jaeger N, Foucher G. Correlation of clinical signs with nerve conduction tests in the diagnosis of carpal tunnel syndrome. J Hand Surg [Br]. 1994;19:720–724.

Buck-Gramko D, Lubahn JD. The Hoffmann––Tinel sign. J Hand Surg. 1993;18B: 800–805.

Campbell DA. How I examine the wrist. Current Orthopaedics. 2001;14:342–346.

De Quervain F. Über eine Form von chronische Tendovaginitis. Correspondez-Nisy G Schweiger Aertze. 1895;25:389–394.

Finkelstein H. Stenosing tendovaginitis at the radial styloid process. J Bone Joint Surg. 1930;12:509.

Forman TA, Forman SK, Rose NE. A clinical approach to diagnosing wrist pain. American Family Physician. 2005;72:1753–1785.

Gelberman RH, Blasingame JP. The timed Allen test. J Trauma. 1981;21:477–479.

Gelberman RH, Eaton R, Urbaniak JR. Peripheral nerve compression. J Bone Joint Surg Am. 1993;75:1854–1878.

Gelmers HJ. The significance of Tinel's sign in the diagnosis of carpal tunnel syndrome. Acta Neurochir. 1979;49:255–258.

Giannini F, Mondelli M, Passero S. Provocative tests in different stages of carpal tunnel syndrome. Clin Neurol Neurosurg. 2001;103:178–183.

Gunnarsson LG, Amilon A, Hellstrand P, Leissner P, Philipson L. The diagnosis of carpal tunnel syndrome: Sensitivity and specificity of some clinical and electrophysiological tests. J Hand Surg [Br]. 1997;22:34–37.

Henderson WR. Clinical assessment of peripheral nerve injuries: Tinel's test. Lancet. 1948;2:801–805.

Hwang JJ, Goldfarb CA, Gelberman RH, Boyer MI. The effect of dorsal carpal ganglion excision on the scaphoid shift test. J Hand Surg [Br]. 1999;24:106–108.

Johnson RP, Carrera GP. Chronic capitolunate instability. J Bone Joint Surg Am.1986;68:1164–1176.

Kanaan N, Sawaya RA. Carpal tunnel syndrome: Modern diagnostic and management techniques. Br J Gen Pract. 2001;51:311–314.

Kuhlman KA, Hennessey WJ. Sensitivity and specificity of carpal tunnel syndrome sings. Am J Phys Med Rehabil. 1997;76:451–457.

Lane LB. The scaphoid shift test. J Hand Surg [Am]. 1993;18:366–368.

LaStayo P, Howell J. Clinical provocative tests used in evaluating wrist pain: A descriptive study. J Hand Ther. 1995;8:10–17.

Mathiowetz V, Weber K, Volland G, Kashman N. Reliability and validity of grip and pinch strength evaluations. J Hand Surg [Am]. 1984;9:222–226.

McConnell EA. Performing Allen's test. Nursing. 1997;27:26.

Murtagh J. De Quervain's tenosynovitis and Finkelstein test. Aust Fam Physician. 1989;18:1552.

Nagle DJ. Evaluation of chronic wrist pain. J Am Acad Orthop Surg. 2000;8:45–55.

Nichols CM, Cheng C. Update on the evaluation of wrist pain. Missouri Medicine. 2006;103:293–296.

Phalen GS. The carpal tunnel syndrome: Seventeen years experience in diagnosis and treatment of six hundred and fifty-four hands. J Bone Joint Surg. 1966;48A:211–228.

Reagan DS, Linscheid RL, Dobyns JH. Lunotriquetral sprains. J Hand Surg [Am]. 1984;9:502–513.

Ruby LK. Carpal instability. J Bone Joint Surg Am. 1995;77:476–487.

Ruby LK, An KN, Linscheid RL, et al. The effect of scapholunate ligament section on scapholunate motion. J Hand Surg [Am]. 1987;12:767–771.

Rush J. De Quervain's disease. Current Orthopaedics. 2000;14:380–383.

Schuett AM, Gieck J, McCue FC. Evaluation and treatment of injuries to the thumb and fingers. Ortop Phys Ther Clin North Am. 1994;3:367–383.

Shin AY, Battaglia MJ, Bishop AT. Lunotriquetral instability: Diagnosis and treatment. J Am Acad Orthop Surg. 2000;8:170–179.

Shin, AY, Battaglia MJ, Bishop, AT. Lunotriquetral instability: Diagnosis and treatment. J Am Acad Orthop Surg. 2000;8:170–179.

Skirven T. Clinical examination of the wrist. J Hand Surg.1996;9:96–107.

Szabo RM, Slater RR Jr, Farver TB, Stanton DB, Sharman WK. The value of diagnostic testing in carpal tunnel syndrome. J Hand Surg [Am]. 1999;24:704–714.

Tetro AM, Evanoff BA, Hollstien SB, Gelberman RH. A new provocative test for carpal tunnel syndrome: Assessment of wrist flexion and nerve compression. J Bone Joint Surg [Br]. 1998;80:493–498.

Thompson CE, Stroud SD. Allen's test: A tool for diagnosing ulnar artery trauma. Nurse Pract. 1984;9:13,16–17.

Wolfe SW, Gupta A, Crisco JJ. Kinematics of the scaphoid shift test. J Hand Surg [Am]. 1997;22:801–806.

## Hip

Asayama I, Naito M, Fujisawa M, Kambe T. Relationship between radiographic measurements of reconstructed hip joint position and the Trendelenburg sign. J Arthroplasty. 2002;17:747–751.

Bartlett MD, Wolf LS, Shurtleff DB, Staheli LT. Hip flexion contractures: A comparison of measurement methods. Arch Phys Med Rehabil. 1985;66:620–625.

Beck M, Kalhor M, Leunig M, Ganz R. Hip morphology influences the pattern of damage to the acetabular cartilage: Femoroacetabular impingement as a cause of early osteoarthritis of the hip. Bone Joint Surg [Br]. 2005;87:1012–1018.

Brady RJ, Dean JB, Skinner TM, Gross MT. Limb length inequality: Clinical implications for assessment and intervention. J Orthop Sports Phys Ther. 2003;33:221–234.

Broadhurst NA, Simmons DN, Bond MJ. Piriformis syndrome: Correlation of muscle morphology with symptoms and signs. Arch Phys Med Rehabil. 2004;85:2036–39.

Dunn DM. Anteversion of the neck of the femur: A method to measurement. J Bone Joint Surg [Br]. 1952;34B:181–186.

Eland DC, Singleton TN, Conaster RR, et al. The "iliacus test:" New information of the evaluation of hip extension dysfunction. J Am Osteopath Assoc. 2002;102:130–142.

Fishman LM, Schaefer MP. The piriformis syndrome is underdiagnosed. Muscle Nerve. 2003;28:646–649.

Fitzgerald RH Jr. Acetabular labrum tears: Diagnosis and treatment. Clin Orthop Relat Res. 1995;311:60–68.

Gabbe BJ, Bennell KL. Reliability of common lower extremity musculoskeletal Screening tests. Physical Therapy in Sport. 2004;5:90–97.

Gajdosik RL, Sandler MM, Marr HL. Influence of knee positions and gender on the Ober test for length of the iliotibial band. Clin Biomech (Bristol, Avon). 2003;18:77–79.

Gautam VK, Anand S. A new test for estimating iliotibial band contracture. Bone Joint Surg [Br]. 1998;80B:474–475.

Hanada E, Kirby RL, Mitchel M, Swuste JM. Measuring leg-length discrepancy by the "iliac crest palpation and book correction" method: Reliability and validity. Arch Phys Med Rehabil. 2001;82:938–942.

Harvey D. Assessment of the flexibility of elite athletes using the modified Thomas test. Br J Sports Med. 1998;32:68–70.

Klaue K, Durnin CW, Ganz R. The acetabular rim syndrome. J Bone Joint Surg [Br]. 1991;73B:423–429.

Kubiak-Langer M, Tannast M, Murphy SB, Siebenrock KA, Langlotz F. Range of motion in anterior femoroacetabular impingement, Clin Orthop, 2007;458:117–124.

Levin U, Nilsson-Wikmar L, Stenstrom CH, Lundeberg T. Reproducibility of manual pressure force on provocation of the sacroiliac joint. Physiother Res Int. 1998;3:1–14.

Margo K, Drezner J, Motzkin D. Evaluation and management of hip pain: An algorithmic approach. J Fam Practice. 2003;52:607–617.

Marks MC, Alexander J, Sutherland DH, Chambers HG. Clinical utility of the Duncan-

Ely test for rectus femoris dysfunction during the swing phase of gait. Dev Med Child Neurol. 2003;45:763–768.

Ober FB. The role of the iliotibial and fascia lata as a factor in the causation of low-back disabilities and sciatica. J Bone Joint Surg. 1936;18:105.

Reynolds D, Lucas J, Klaue K. Retroversion of the acetabulum. J Bone Joint Surg. 1999;81B:281–288.

Robroy L, Martin PT, Keelan R, et al. Acetabular labral tears of the hip: Examination and diagnostic challenges. J Orthop Sports Phys Ther. 2006;36:503–515.

Ross MD, Nordeen MH, Barido M. Test-retest reliability of Patrick's hip range of motion test in healthy college-aged men. J Strength Cond Res. 2003;17:156–161.

Ruwe PA, Yage JR, Ozonoff MB, De Luca PA. Clinical determination of femoral anteversion: A comparison with established techniques. J Bone Joint Surg [Am]. 1992;74:820–830.

Ryder CT, Crane L. Measuring femoral anteversion: The problem and a method. J Bone Joint Surg [Am]. 1953;35A:321–328.

Scopp JM, Moormann CT. The assessment of athletic hip injury. Clin Sports Med. 2001;20:647–659.

Stewart JD. The Piriformis syndrome is over-diagnosed. Muscle Nerve. 2003;28:644–646.

Stone M, Ellis D. How I examine the hip. Current Orthopaedics. 2000;14:262–266.

Tönnis D, Heinecke A. Acetabular and femoral anteversion: Relationship with osteoarthritis of the hip. J Bone Joint Surg. 1999;81A:1747–1768.

Trendelenburg F. Trendelenburg's test: 1895. Clin Orthop Relat Res. 1998;355:3–7.

van der Wurff P, Meyne W, Hagmeijer RH. Clinical tests of the sacroiliac joint: A systemic methodological review;Part 1: Reliability. Man Ther. 2000;5:30–36.

van der Wurff P, Meyne W, Hagemeijer RH. Clinical tests of the sacroiliac joint. Man Ther. 2000;5:89–96.

Vasudevan PN, Vaidyalingam KV, Nair PB. Can Trendelenburg's sign be positive if the hip is normal? J Bone Joint Surg [Br]. 1997;79:462–466.

# Knee

Anderson AF, Lipscomb AB. Clinical diagnosis of meniscal tears: Description of a new manipulative test. Am J Sports Med. 1986;14:291–293.

Anderson AF, Renniert GW, Standeffer WC Jr. Clinical analysis of the pivot shift tests: Description of the pivot drawer test. Am J Knee Surg. 2000;13:19–23.

Apley AG. The diagnosis of meniscus injuries. J Bone Joint Surg. 1947;29:78–84.

Bahk MS, Cosgarea AJ. Physical examination and imaging of the lateral collateral ligament and posterolateral corner of the knee. Sports Med Arthrose Rev. 2006;14:12–19.

Biedert RM, Warnke K. Correlation between the Q angle and the patella position: A clinical and axial computed tomography evaluation. Arch Orthop Trauma Surg. 2001;121:346–349.

Bollen S. How I examine the knee. Current Orthopaedics. 2000;14:189–192.

Caylor D, Fites R, Worrell TW. The relationship between quadriceps angle and anterior knee pain syndrome. J Orthop Sports Phys Ther. 1993;17:11–16.

Cooperman JM, Riddle DL, Rothstein JM. Reliability and validity of judgments of the integrity of the ACL of the knee using the Lachman's test. Phys Ther. 1990;70:225–233.

Dimon JH. Apprehension test for subluxation of the patella. Clin Orthop Relat Res. 1974;103:39.

Dupont JY, Bellier G. The jerk-test in external rotation in rupture of the anterior cruciate ligament: Description and significance. Rev Chir Orthop Reparat Appar Mot. 1988;74:413–423.

Eren OT. The accuracy of joint line tenderness by physical examination in the diagnosis of meniscal teras. The Journal of Arthroscopic Related Surgery. 2003;19:850–854.

Evans PJ, Bell GD, Frank C. Prospective evaluation of the McMurray test. Am J Sports Med. 1993;21:604–608.

Fanelli GCF, Orcutt DR, Edson CFE. The multiple-ligament injured knee: Evaluation, treatment, and results. The Journal of Arthroscopic and Related Surgery. 2005;21:471–486.

Fowler PJ, Lubliner JA. The predictive value of five clinical signs in the evaluation of meniscal pathology. Arthroscopy. 1989;5:184–186.

Fredericson M, Yoon K. Physical examination and patellofemoral pain syndrome. Am J Phys Med Rehabil. 2006;85:234–243.

Fulkerson JP. Diagnosis and treatment of patients with patellofemoral pain. Am J Sports Med. 2002;30:447–456.

Galway RD, Beaupre A, Macintosh DL. Pivot shift. J Bone Joint Surg [Br]. 1972;54:763.

Gose JC, Schweizer P. Iliotibial band tightness. J Orthop Sports Phys Ther. 1989;10:399–407.

Greene CC, Edwards TB, Wade MR, et al. Reliability of the quadriceps angle measurement. Am J Knee Surg. 2001;14:97–103.

Herrington L, Nester C. Q-angle undervalued? The relationship between Q-angle and medio-lateral position of the patella. Clin Biomech (Bristol, Avon). 2004;19:1070–1073.

Hughston JC. The absent posterior drawer test in some acute posterior cruciate ligament tears of the knee. Am J Sports Med. 1988;16:39–43.

Hughston JC, Norwood LA Jr. The posterolateral drawer test and external rotational recurvatum test for posterolateral rotatory instability of the knee. Clin Orthop Relat Res. 1980;147:82–87.

Hvid I, Andersen LI. The quadriceps angle and its relation to femoral torsion. Acta Orthop Scand. 1982;53:577–579.

Jakob RP, Hassler H, Staebuli HU. Observations on rotary instability of the lateral compartment of the knee. Acta Orthop Scand Suppl. 1981;52:1–32.

Jerosch J, Rieber S. How good are clinical investigative procedures for diagnosing meniscus lesions? Sportverletz Sportschaden. 2004;18:59–67.

Johnson MW. Acute knee effusions: A systematic approach to diagnosis. Am Fam Physician. 2000;61:2391–2400.

Jonsson T, Althoff B, Peterson L, Renstrom P. Clinical diagnosis of ruptures of the anterior cruciate ligament: A comparative study of the Lachman's test and the anterior drawer sign. Am J Sports Med. 1982;10:100.

Kannus P, Natri A, Paakkala T, et al. An outcome study of chronic patellofemoral pain syndrome: Seven-year follow-up of patients in a randomized, controlled trial. J Bone Joint Surg [Am]. 1999;81:355–363.

Kim SJ, Kim HK. Reliability of the anterior drawer test, the pivot shift test, and the Lachman test. Clin Orthop Relat Res. 1995;319:237–242.

König DP, Rutt J, Kumm D, Breidenbach E. Diagnosis of anterior knee instability: Comparison between the Lachman test, the KT-1,000 arthrometer and the ultrasound Lachman test. Unfallchirurg. 1998;101:209–213.

Kumar AJ, Bickerstaff D. Posterolateral instability of the knee. Current Orthopaedics. 2000;14:337–341.

LaPrade RF, Wentorf F. Diagnosis and treatment of posterolateral knee injuries. Clin Orthop Relat Res. 2002;402:110–121.

Lin YC, Davey C, Cochrane T. Tests for physical function of the elderly with knee and hip osteoarthritis. Scand J Med Sci Sports. 2001;11:280–286.

Livingston LA. The accuracy of Q angle values. Clin Biomech (Bristol, Avon). 2002;17:322–324.

Logan M, Williams A, Lavelle J, Gedroyc W, Freeman M. The effect of posterior cruciate ligament deficiency on knee kinematics. Am J Sports Med. 2004;32:1915–1922.

Loomer RL. A test for knee posterolateral rotatory instability. Clin Orthop Relat Res. 1991;264:235–238.

Malanga GA, Andrus S, Nadler SF, McLean J. Physical examination of the knee: A review of the original test description and scientific validity of common orthopaedic tests. Ach Phys Med Rehabil. 2003;84:592–603.

McMurray TP. The semilunar cartilages. Br J Surg. 1942;29:407–414.

Miller MD, Berfeld JA. The posterior cruciate ligament injured knee: Principles of evaluation and treatment. AAOS Instr Course Lect. 1999;48:199–207.

Olerud C, Berg P. The variation of the Q angle with different positions of the foot. Clin Orthop Relat Res. 1984;191:162–165.

Orndorff DG, Hart JA, Miller MD. Physical Examination of the Knee. Current Sports Medicine Reports. 2005;4:243–248.

Quarles JD, Hosey RG. Medial and lateral collateral injuries: Prognosis and treatment. Prim Care. 2004;31:957–975.

Sandler DA. Homan's sign and medical education. Lancet. 1985;2:1130–1131.

Scholten RJ, Devillé WL, Opstelten W, Bijl D, Van der Plas CG, Bouter LM. The accuracy of physical diagnostic tests of assessing meniscal lesions of the knee: Meta-analysis. J Fam Pract. 2001;50:938–944.

Shino K, Mitsuoka T, Horibe S, Hamada M, Nakata K, Nakamura N. The gravity sag view: A simple radiographic technique to show posterior laxity of the knee. Arthroscopy. 2000;16:670–672.

Slocum DB, James SL, Larson RL, Singer KM. Clinical test for anterolateral rotary instability of the knee. Clin Orthop. 1976;118:63–69.

Slocum DB, Larson RL. Rotatory instability of the knee. J Bone Joint Surg [Am]. 1968;50:211–225.

Staubli HU, Jakob RP. Posterior instability of the knee near extension: A clinical and stress radiographic analysis of acute injuries of the posterior cruciate ligament. J Bone Joint Surg [Br]. 1990;72:225–230.

Strobel MJ, Weiler A, Schulz MS, Russe K, Eichhorn HJ. Fixed posterior subluxation in posterior cruciate ligament-deficient knees: Diagnosis and treatment of a new clinical sign. Am J Sports Med. 2002;30:32–38.

Tegner Y, Lysholm J. Rating systems in the evaluation of knee ligament injuries. Clin Orthop. 1985;198:43–49.

Winslow J, Yoder E. Patellofemoral pain in female ballet dancers: Correlation with iliotibial band tightness and tibial external rotation. J Orthop Sports Phys Ther. 1995;22:18–21.

## Ankle and Foot

Alonso A, Khoury L, Adams R. Clinical tests for ankle syndesmosis injury: Reliability and prediction of return to function. J Orthop Sports Phys Ther. 1998;27:276–284.

Bahr R, Pena F, Shine J, et al. Mechanics of the anterior drawer and talar tilt tests. Acta Orthop Scand. 1997;68:435–441.

Bailie DS, Kelikian AS. Tarsal tunnel syndrome: Diagnosis, surgical technique, and functional outcome. Foot Ankle Int. 1998;19:65–72.

Beumer A, Swierstra BA, Mulder PGH. Clinical diagnosis of syndesmotic ankle instability. Acta Orthop Scand. 2002;73:667–669.

Beumer A, van Hemmert WL, Swierstra BA, Jasper LE, Belkoff SM. A biomechanical evaluation of clinical stress tests for syndesmotic ankle instability. Foot Ankle Int. 2003;24:358–363.

Burns B, Maffuli N. Lower limb injuries in children in sports. Clin Sports Med. 2000;19:637–662.

Cloke DJ, Greiss ME. The digital nerve stretch test: A sensitive indicator of Morton's neuroma and neuritis. Foot and Ankle Surgery. 2006;12:201–203.

Gaebler C, Kukla C, Breitenseher MJ, et al. Diagnosis of lateral ankle ligament injuries. Acta Ortop Scand. 1997;68:286–290.

Hamilton WG, Geppert MJ, Thompson FM. Pain in the posterior aspect of the ankle in dancers: Differential diagnosis and operative treatment. J Bone Joint Surg [Am]. 1996;78:1491–1500.

Hedrick MR, McBryde Am. Posteriore ankle impingement. Foot Ankle Int. 1994;15:2–8.

Hopkinson WJ, St. Pierre P, Ryan JB, Wheeler JH. Syndesmosis sprains of the ankle. Foot Ankle Int. 1990;10:325–330.

Kinoshita M, Okuda R, Morikawa J. Jotoku T, Abe M. The dorsiflexion-eversion test for diagnosis of tarsal tunnel syndrome. J Bone Joint Surg. 2001;83A:1935–1939.

Kleiger B. Anterior tibiotalar impingement syndromes in dancers. Foot Ankle Int. 1983;3:69–73.

Klenerman L. How I examine the foot. Current Orthopaedics. 2001;15:152–155.

Lin CF, Gross MT, Weinhold P. Ankle syndesmosis injuries: Anatomy, biomechanics, mechanism of injury, and clinical guidelines for diagnosis and intervention. J Orthop Sports Phys Ther. 2006;36:372–384.

Liu SH, Jason WJ. Lateral ankle sprains and instability problems. Clin Sports Med. 1994;13:793–809.

Liu W, Maitland ME, Nigg BM. The effect of axial load on the in vivo anterior drawer test of the ankle joint complex. Foot Ankle Int. 2000;21:420–426.

Marotta JJ, Micheli LJ. Os trigonum impingement in dancers. Am J Sports Med. 1992;20:533–536.

Ray RG, Christensen JC, Gusman DN. Critical evaluation of anterior drawer measurement methods in the ankle. Clin Orthop. 1997;334:215–224.

Shookster L, Falke G, Ducic I, Maloney C Jr, Dellon A. Fibromyalgia and Tinel's sign in the foot. J Am Podiatr Med Assoc. 2004;94:400–403.

Sizer PS Jr, Phelps V, Dedrick G, James R, Matthijs O. Diagnosis and management of the painful ankle/foot, Part 2: Examination, interpretation, and management. Pain Practice. 2003;3:343–374.

Stamatis ED, Karabalis C. Interdigital neuromas: Current state of the art-surgical. Foot Ankle Int. 2004;25:287–296.

Thompson TC. A test for rupture of the tendo achillis. Acta Orthop Scand. 1962;32:461–465.

Tohyama H, Yasuda K, Ohkoshi Y, et al. Anterior drawer test for acute anterior talofibular ligament injuries of the ankle: How much load should be applied during the test? Am J Sports Med. 2003;31:226–232.

Tol JL, van Dijk CN. Etiology of the anterior ankle impingement syndrome: A descriptive anatomical study. Foot Ankle Int. 2004;25:382–386.

Tol JL, Verhagen RA, Krips R, et al. The anterior ankle impingement syndrome: Diagnostic value of oblique radiographs. Foot Ankle Int. 2004;25:63–68.

van Dijk, CN. Anterior and posterior ankle impingement. Foot Ankle Clin N Am. 2006;11:663–683.

van Dijk, CN, Lim LS, Poortmann A, et al. Degenerative joint disease in female ballet dancers. Am J Sports Med. 1995;23:295–300.

van Dijk, CN, Mol BWJ, Lim LS, Marti RK, Bossuyt PMM. Diagnosis of ligament rupture of the ankle joint. Acta Orthop Scand. 1996;67:566–570.

Young CC, Niedfeldt MW, Morris GA, Eerkes, KJ. Clinical examination of the foot and ankle. Prim Care Clin Office Pract. 2005;32:105–132.

## Posture Deficiency

Fialka-Moser V, Uher EM, Lack W. Postural disorders in children and adolescents. Wien Med Wochenschr. 1994;144:577–592.

Mahlknecht JF. Die Prävalenz von Haltungsstörungen bei Kindern und Jugendlichen: Eine Querschnittsanalyse. Z Orthop Unfallchir. 2007;145:338–342.

Widhe T. Spine: Posture, mobility and pain;A longitudinal study from childhood to adolescence. Eur Spine J. 2001;10:118–123.

## Occlusive Arterial Disease— Venous Thrombosis

Allen EV. Thromboangiitis obliterans: Methods of diagnosis of chronic occlusive arterial lesions distal to the wrist with illustrative case. Am J Med Sci. 1929;178:237–244.

Allen EV, Brown GE. Raynaud's desease affecting men. Ann Intern Med. 1932;5:1384–1386.

Cranley JJ, Canos AJ, Sull WJ. The diagnosis of deep venous thrombosis: Fallibility of clinical symptoms and signs. Arch Surg. 1976;111:34–36.

Kim J, Richards S, Kent PJ. Clinical examination of varicose veins: A validation study. Annals of the Royal College of Surgeons of England. 2000;82:171–175.

McConnell EA. Performing Allen's test. Nursing. 1997;21:26.

Stober R. Das Thoracic-outlet-Syndrom. (Schweiz). Rundschau Med. 1989;78:1063–1070.

Wenz W, Rahmanzadeh M, Husfeldt KJ. Das neurovaskuläre Kompressionssyndrom der oberen Thoraxappertur: Eine wichtige Differentialdiagnose für Beschwerden im Bereich der oberen Extremität. Deutsches Ärzteblatt. 1998;95(13):S. A/736–B/596–C/561.

# Index